Praise for Paola's Writing

Paola's writing is vivid and extremely readable. She has an eye for the unusual and the moving detail. I read her work with great pleasure and interest.
Alexander McCall Smith

Paola's writing is colourful, exact and perceptive, and she has a keen eye for the unusual and the easily overlooked. I can't recommend her too highly.
Jeremy Lewis, *The Oldie*

I loved it and was very moved: it reminds me of Gerald Durrell's My Family and Other Animals.
Brigid Keenan, author of *Diplomatic Baggage*

A well-travelled and keen observer, Paola writes with wit and inspiring respect for the diversity of humanity.
Christopher Allen, author of *Other Household Toxins*

I will never forget the snake on the train; I can still SEE it!
Sister Mary Germaine O'Neill, IBVM

Leap
Into the
Light

Paola Fornari Hanna

Copyright © 2022 Paola Fornari Hanna

The moral right of the author has been asserted.

Apart from any fair dealing for the purposes of research or private study, or criticism or review, as permitted under the Copyright, Designs and Patents Act 1988, this publication may only be reproduced, stored or transmitted, in any form or by any means, with the prior permission in writing of the publishers, or in the case of reprographic reproduction in accordance with the terms of licences issued by the Copyright Licensing Agency. Enquiries concerning reproduction outside those terms should be sent to the publishers.

Cover photo: Cousin Vari's house, Urambo, Tanganyika

Matador
Unit E2 Airfield Business Park,
Harrison Road, Market Harborough,
Leicestershire. LE16 7UL
Tel: 0116 2792299
Email: books@troubador.co.uk
Web: www.troubador.co.uk/matador
Twitter: @matadorbooks

ISBN 978 1803135 427

British Library Cataloguing in Publication Data.
A catalogue record for this book is available from the British Library.

Printed on FSC accredited paper
Printed and bound in Great Britain by 4edge Limited
Typeset in 11pt Minion Pro by Troubador Publishing Ltd, Leicester, UK

Matador is an imprint of Troubador Publishing Ltd

I dedicate this book to my brother Enrico and my sister Silvia who have accompanied me from the night I was born under the African stars on Ukerewe Island to this day.

Contents

Preface	xi
Abbateggio, Abruzzo: 1947–1951	1
The Springboard	3
Life Before Life	7
The Madonna, Magic, and Medicine	10
Light Years Distant	14
Urambo, Tanganyika: March–May 1951	17
The Telegram	19
Ukerewe: 1951–1954	25
Paradise Island	27
Medical Matters	36
The Ugly Baby	43
Rome: July–November 1954	49
Long Leave	51
Musoma: 1954–1957	55
Musoma Memories	57

Bromley, Kent: 1957–1958	**63**
Smog	65
Letters from Bromley	**71**
Kigoma: 1958–1961	**77**
The Kaiserhof	79
Trains, Boats, and a Ferry	83
In the Doctor's Footsteps	88
Christmas in Kigoma	91
Lake Tanganyika	95
Like Lions	99
Kingdoms of Sand	104
Nairobi and Mwanza: 1961–1963	**109**
A Speck of Dust	111
Blending In	116
Rituals and Illness	121
An Antelope and Other Creatures	127
Crimson and Scarlet	133
The Secret	139
Speedy Gonzales	144
Edinburgh: 1963–1964	**147**
Spaghetti's the Only Veg	149
Dar es Salaam and Nairobi: 1964–1966	**155**
Haven of Peace	157
Playing the Part	163
Nerone	169

Nairobi and Dar es Salaam: 1967–1972   **173**
The World Beyond   175
Teenagers and Tek-Teks   181
Champagne Socialism   186
What Lies Beneath   191
'A' Level Years   196
Pauline and the Pool   201

Kilimanjaro: 1972–2001   **207**
Uhuru   209

Edinburgh: 1973–1974   **217**
The Yellow Brick Road   219

Rome: November 2021   **225**
Closure   227

Glossary   **233**
Acknowledgements   **235**
References   **237**

Preface

I was born on an island on Lake Victoria, and grew up in Tanganyika, which later became Tanzania. My father, a doctor, worked there for thirty-four years. This book recounts what it was like growing up in an Italian family in pre- and post-colonial East Africa.

During lockdown in 2021, I started writing my story in a blog. It seemed right to begin in Italy with my father's first experience as a doctor in the remote town of Abbateggio in Abruzzo. During his retirement, reminiscing about those days, my father wrote:

In 1935, for Carlo Levi, doctor, painter and writer, Christ had only reached Eboli; he had stopped short of the backward, desperate village in Lucania where Levi was exiled for his anti-fascist views. Fifteen years later, for Maria and me, Christ had only reached San Valentino d'Abruzzo; he had stopped short of Abbateggio. In retrospect, three and a half years of medical practice in a remote town near the Maiella, in a house with no bathroom, no running water, and no heating, turned out to be what we called our first African experience, in conditions almost identical to those described by Levi in Christ Stopped at Eboli. *What mysterious moral force helped us to live happily in such squalor?*

My father took hundreds of black and white photos and printed them in makeshift darkrooms over the years. When he retired, he sent fresh copies to us, and he and my mother wrote to us, recalling those times.

As I wrote my blog, many people got in touch: relatives, friends and colleagues who had known my parents in Abruzzo and Tanganyika, boarding school friends, and complete strangers, sharing memories which my account had triggered.

My mother died in 2018, and my father in 2021. In their apartment in Rome, I came across a shoebox filled with vivid letters, written mostly by my mother to her parents in the 1950s, starting from before I was born and before my earliest memories. I have included some extracts. All translations are mine.

This book is a mosaic of my own imperfect memories, letters, photos, family folklore, and people and their stories; people who were there before me, those who travelled along the way with me, and those who made me into who I am.

Most characters are real, but, especially in the school chapters, some are a mixture of several people, and I have changed some names. I have tried to give an impression of how we saw our world at that time, without judgment.

I regret not having asked my parents and grandparents more about their lives, experiences, and feelings. I hope this account will answer some of the questions my children and grandchildren may have about my childhood and upbringing. Writing it has helped me with my quest for an answer to the question I am often asked: 'Where are you from?' I hope the book does the same for them.

ABBATEGGIO, ABRUZZO

1947-1951

The Springboard

I was perpetually astonished to see cases that any good doctor would have branded as hopeless improve and recover with the simplest kind of care. Carlo Levi: *Christ Stopped at Eboli.*

In October 1947, a man travelled by rickety truck a hundred and eighty-five kilometres east from his home city of Rome to the town of Abbateggio in the mountains of Abruzzo. His journey was hampered by rain, fog, and slippery roads. He was the second eldest of seven children, and was keen to help his family by becoming independent as quickly as possible. At twenty-three, having skipped two years at school, he was the youngest medical graduate of his year. He would not have chosen to come to such a desolate place, far from his family and fiancée, but he accepted the first job offered to him.

That new doctor was my father, Ugo Fornari.

His younger sister Teta, a nurse, accompanied him, to assist him in his work and help him settle in his new home.

Two days after their arrival, she wrote home.

Abbateggio, October 31st, 1947

Dear family,

We're coming to the end of our second day in this illustrious district. All well. There has been so much work, and so many people coming to meet 'u 'gnor dottò' [Mr. Doctor Sir], that we haven't had a moment to look around. Poor Ugo! He must have examined and treated twenty people. Now he's removing an upper molar from a fellow who's sitting in the middle of this empty room; the tools are laid out on two chairs. May God look after them both because Ugo has realised he has neither the right forceps, nor any Novocaine for the anaesthetic. The tooth is out now, painlessly.

A short while ago we visited a woman who looked as though she was about to miscarry, and she probably had ovarian cysts too, and before that a young girl with a deep gash in her leg (we had to accept two grappas and two disgusting coffees, so as not to offend).

Back to the beginning: Ugo would be outraged if my letter didn't cover everything from 2.20 a.m. of Thursday 30th October.

We left Rome in a hurry. The driver seemed quite relaxed as he sped along at 80 kph. We arrived in Pescara at eight, with enough rain to wash not just that small town, but half the world, dirty as it is. At Pescara, a quick snack in a bar, while the truck waited outside to bring us here (we'd already agreed with the driver to pay the modest sum of 1,500 lire). Since we were only expected towards evening (and it was ten in the morning), they were still cleaning the house, so we went to our landlords, who invited us to lunch.

Straight after lunch, we set to work. In a few hours, everything was tidy, apart from the surgery, which was still in chaos.

At eight we went to bed and slept straight through till seven this morning. I forgot to mention that towards evening the sky cleared, and this morning the beautiful valley surrounding Abbateggio was bathed in magnificent sunshine. The house is well exposed; sunlight comes in from everywhere, when it's there. However, this evening it's raining again. After six days of rain the mud is dreadful, and the roads are chaotic because they're putting in water pipes.

Help! I've just opened the door to another patient who needs his tooth removed. We'll end up having dinner at nine tonight. Speaking of food, we're doing rather well. Summary of gifts received (in exchange for services, of course): ½ kilo walnuts, 3 kilos apples, ½ kilo pasta or maybe more, a loaf of bread, a focaccia, 7 eggs, a jar of tomato preserve, and a little salt.

Tomorrow I will find a woman to bring water and to wash the clothes when necessary.

The people here are so helpful. The landlady comes around all the time to ask whether we need anything: she brings water, but would like to do more. She's rough but kind and good. Yesterday two young girls came to bring some things that Ugo had ordered, and they insisted on sweeping the house. Since I was unpacking, they marvelled at every lovely object that appeared from those magical boxes.

Now I have no more space, but tomorrow I'll write again. Infinite thanks to all of you for what you've done for us, especially mamma and papá. We're very well: what about you?

Lots of love,
Teta and Ugo

*

Abbateggio is situated near the Maiella massif in the Central Apennines. Today, fewer than 400 people live there. In my father's day, its population numbered about 1,500, half of whom lived in the town, and the rest in surrounding hamlets. During harsh winters, it was snowbound for long periods.

The land was rugged and poor, and the people eked out their existence by keeping a few chickens and goats. A fountain was the only source of water. There were no phones, and the electricity supply was erratic. People travelled by mule. Only the priest, the teacher, and now the doctor, had an inside toilet. There was a bar, where the men went after work. A small shop, where sheep were butchered on Saturdays, provided basic necessities.

Looking back on this period many years later, my father wrote:

I arrived in Abbateggio at the tender age of twenty-three and a half, as soon as I had been granted my professional licence, so that I could quickly become independent and begin to live with mamma as soon as possible. When I arrived, many people didn't believe that a youngster like me could be a graduate, but they soon got used to the idea. It was a sad and desolate place, which, however, I (and later mamma, when she joined me) saw through eyes and a spirit filled with trust and enthusiasm. Life there was tough, there was certainly no shortage of work, and there was hardship. I always say that mamma and I had our first 'African' experience in Abbateggio, which then became our springboard towards the real African adventure.

Life Before Life

> *The women supplicated me, calling down blessings on my head and kissing my hands. Their faith and hope in me were absolute and I could only wonder at them.* Carlo Levi: *Christ Stopped at Eboli.*

Abbateggio had never had a doctor before. The townspeople welcomed my father as a saviour, with unconditional trust, respect, and admiration.

He was assigned a house with four bedrooms, two of which were set up as a consulting room and a surgery. For emergencies, he had to travel across rocky hillsides, often through mud or snow, to his patients' homes, to attend to the sick, or deliver a baby.

When the people came to call me, he wrote, *they'd ask if I wanted 'the mount', which was a mule. I only rode it two or three times, because I preferred to get around on foot. Sometimes I even ran, so the local people began to call me 'lu dottore piu' corridore del contorno'* [the fastest running doctor in the area].

His patients were scattered over the hillsides, and on occasion, when a labour took longer than expected, my father would snuggle up in the only bed in the house with the expectant parents to get some rest.

In April 1948, the time came for my father to get married in Rome. He had known my mother for several years: his sister Lolli and she had been good friends at school.

Before he left Abbateggio for the wedding, he appointed Orsolina, a bright young war widow with two small children, to look after his practice. He taught her to give injections and dress wounds.

My parents' wedding was a small and modest occasion. My father wore a pinstriped double-breasted suit. My mother's powder-blue wedding dress was simple, flared from the waist, the bodice decorated with bows. It reached just below the knee, as was the fashion just after the war. A light matching coat protected her from the spring chill.

After a short honeymoon in Capri, my mother got her first sight of Abbateggio.

She was nineteen, the middle child of a well-to-do family. She had never before lacked material comforts. But she was madly in love and ready to follow her young doctor to the ends of the earth. Perhaps the fact that her home environment had been rigid made it easier for her to leave.

Orsolina had done well as locum, but the patients had missed their doctor, and gave my father and his young bride a warm welcome.

In Abbateggio, eggs symbolised fertility. The townspeople offered my mother so many eggs that she didn't know what to do with them: my parents ate three for lunch and three for dinner every day, and she sent a caseful to her mother-in-law in Rome, but there were still plenty left over.

A woman called Filomena helped around the house, cleaned, and fetched water from the well.

'Sell the eggs,' Filomena said, but my mother felt she could hardly dispose of such kindness in this way.

'Give them to my mother who will sell them,' Filomena suggested, 'then you can buy a pig with the earnings. That way when you have a baby he will not lack food.'

It seemed a good idea, but my mother did not fancy keeping a pig on her terrace. A deal was done, the pig was bought, and Filomena's mother kept it at her home, in exchange for half of it when the time came for the slaughter. It was fed on scraps from the doctor's table, and the overflow of patients' gifts.

Abbateggio, my father wrote, *marked an important stage in my life and mamma's, a stage in which we started walking together in this strange life – a mysterious and incredible journey. Although Paola was not physically with us, and I could say the same about Enrico and Silvia before they were born, in some ways she was there, even if mamma and I hadn't found her yet. Sometimes it is said that someone who is born or something that happens were 'in mente Dei'* [in the mind of God], *before that somebody was born or that something happened. But I like to think – even if this is an absurd and inexplicable concept – that Enrico, Silvia and Paola were already there 'before'. It was mamma and I who found them and took them with us and made them a part of us, in the same way as Mozart found* Symphony No. 40 in G Minor, *or Michelangelo discovered* The Last Judgment, *which already existed, floating about somewhere from time immemorial.*

This philosophy was not unique in my father's family: when she was well into her eighties and frail, but mentally still sharp, his sister Lolli said to me, 'You know, Paola, I'm not afraid of dying. Imagine going back to that wonderfully peaceful place you were in, for ever, before you were born! How comforting!'

The Madonna, Magic, and Medicine

> *... magic... was harmless enough, and the peasants considered it in no way in conflict with official medicine.* Carlo Levi: *Christ Stopped at Eboli.*

My parents complemented each other: my father was introverted, perhaps even ascetic, meticulous. My mother was sociable and fun-loving, embracing everything that was new.

She soon adapted to her new role as wife of the respected doctor, and turned out to be an excellent assistant. Patients did not pay for consultations, as my father received a small stipend from the local administration. But they always offered her *il cumplimento per la signora*: gifts of oil, wine, goat's cheese, eggs, and seasonal fruit and vegetables.

Although she was originally from Chiavenna, a town in the north of Italy, near the Swiss border, my mother learnt the local dialect quickly. The people found her amenable, and often consulted her first, opening their hearts to her, telling her about a stomach 'fire' or a chest 'rattle'. She would then relay the information to my father. 'The baby's pushing up instead of down,' a woman once told her, 'so it's not coming out!'

Superstition and religion were interwoven in the local culture. A woman who had caught a cold in April consulted my father: 'Perhaps it's because I washed my feet too soon after the winter,' she said. In fact, custom had it that a full bath was taken only three times: the first at birth, the second before marriage, and the third before burial.

Traditionally, newlyweds' linen sheets were paraded through the streets the morning after a wedding... many a hen was sacrificed to preserve the bride's honour. Since my parents were not married in the town, they were spared this ignominy.

I recall, my father wrote, *that it was not unusual, in difficult cases, especially with sick children, for people to turn simultaneously to me, to the* magaro *who would mix potions and recite incantations to exorcise the patient, and to the miraculous Madonna dell'Elcina, with whom the people tried to ingratiate themselves by pinning banknotes onto the fabric of the cape her statue wore.*

The Madonna dell'Elcina was, and still is, the town's protectress. Oral legend dating back to the fifteenth or sixteenth century has it that in times gone by two mute shepherd boys tending their sheep on a hillside saw an apparition of the Virgin Mary sitting in an oak tree, with the Christ child in her arms. At the foot of the tree stood an image of the scene they were witnessing: a picture of the Madonna and child in the tree.

'Build a church over on that hill,' the Madonna said to them. The boys ran home, and spoke for the first time in their lives, telling their mother what had happened. The news spread in the neighbourhood, and people flocked to the site. Although the young shepherd boys could still see the Madonna, all that was visible to the onlookers was the image. Three times, the image was taken by the faithful to the local church of San Lorenzo, but each time it miraculously reappeared under the tree. A chapel was built at the site.

My father didn't mind who got credit for a recovery: this teamwork between medicine, religion and witchcraft seemed to work, and to satisfy the people.

He wrote: *They thought that in serious cases, every force, including myself, shared responsibility for the case and merit for the cure.*

In May, a month after my parents' wedding, my mother became pregnant. In November the pig that had been bought with the proceeds of the eggs was slaughtered, and rows of salamis and prosciuttos were hung in the kitchen for curing. When my father delivered my brother Enrico at home in mid-February, there was enough food for a party for the whole town, and plenty left over.

Enrico thrived. Before he was a year old, he learnt to walk on the terrace, surprising my mother, who once just managed to catch him as he was about to step over the edge.

Just under two years after Enrico's birth, in mid-January, my sister Silvia was born. My mother was in the pharmacy in San Valentino, three and a half kilometres down the hill, when labour set in. 'You'd better go home,' the pharmacist, Don Camillo, said, and my mother trudged all the way back up the mountain through the snow. Once again, they were alone in their home for the delivery. It was night-time when things began to move quickly. My mother kept nudging my father. 'I think it's time!' but he rolled over and went back to sleep. Finally, at five in the morning, she could bear it no longer. 'The baby is here!' He got up just in time. 'What a lot of hair!' he exclaimed, as Silvia came into the world.

My father's new role was not easy. He wrote: *We lived in a place where the people, albeit ignorant and primitive, loved us deeply. With their genuine affection, they helped us overcome the many difficulties we had to face: among these the greatest was my professional inexperience, which initially caused me great anxiety. A newly graduated doctor knows little about medicine, and if you have a sense of responsibility and a character like mine, you are all the more aware of this. I still tremble when I think back to the many difficult cases I had to tackle, which I was not always able to solve satisfactorily, especially in the field of obstetrics.*

In a place so isolated from the civilised world, particularly when we were cut off by the snow in mid-winter, it was difficult to get advice from more experienced doctors. Today I am amazed that I took on the serious responsibility of assisting mamma single-handed when Enrico and Silvia were born. Fortunately, both times it went well (as it did when Paola was born three years later in Kagunguli, when at least I had a bit more experience).

Retrospectively, I can't help but think that all three times it was presumptuous on my part to have wanted to manage on my own, without asking for assistance from someone who could have shared the burden with me. In hindsight we could say that this is the way it had to be, and mamma and I are happy to have managed on our own.

Light Years Distant

But what have we to hope for... This is no place to live. A man must get away. Now we are going to Africa. It's our last chance. Carlo Levi: *Christ Stopped at Eboli.*

As children, we spent many hours in my father's improvised darkrooms in the various houses where we lived. We watched, transfixed, as perfect reproductions of people and scenes miraculously appeared in black and white on glossy blank sheets soaking in developing fluid, reaching just the right point of contrast before they were transferred to the fixing liquid.

Today, pictures from our past still emerge, like images forming on blank sheets.

In January 2021, I spoke to Cristina DeThomasis, a woman who had emigrated from Abbateggio in her late teens. I contacted her via her daughter, whom I had met on a trip to Abbateggio. The Italian voice on the line, all the way from Albany, New York, with its strong Abruzzo accent, was affable and clear. I felt as though she was in the room with me, and we chatted like old friends. Well into her eighties, Cristina's memory was sharp, and her nostalgia for her hometown palpable.

'I was about ten years old,' she said, 'when your father arrived in the town. We were all so happy. We'd never had our own doctor before: we had to go to San Valentino if we needed one. Dottor Ugo used to stop by at our house for a coffee and a chat. My mother would give him fresh ricotta. I remember your mother, too, and your brother, in his pram, on that big terrace.

'One evening, my brother, who was thirteen, rode our pregnant donkey to the fountain, which was the only water supply we had. Dusk was setting in. On the way home, the donkey lost her footing and slipped into a gully, landing on the jagged branch of a tree. My brother was unscathed, but the donkey was seriously injured: she had a deep gash on her stomach. Your father was called – we had no vet – and he sewed her up. The foal was born safely a month later.

'Oh, we missed them so much when they left. My family emigrated to the United States, too, some years later, and I married an Abbateggio man. Many people were driven away, back then. Times were hard. I will never forget your father. He saved our donkey's life.'

'Do you remember the donkey you rescued?' I asked my father, not long before he died. He hesitated. I told him the story.

'I remember,' he said, after a long pause.

He was more expansive in the letters he sent us, along with reprinted photos, in 1992.

There's so much to say about our life in Abbateggio, he wrote. *Mamma will add some of her memories, to help you understand how she too found happiness in a place that was so poor and desolate.*

My mother's writing style was much chattier, more direct, less formal.

When Enrico and Silvia were born, she wrote, *every family in the town brought me a chicken. According to tradition, I should have eaten just the broth and the neck, and papà the rest. When a baby was born, mother and child had to stay cooped up in the bedroom for forty days, after which they could emerge, all dressed up, for the baptism. Fortunately, we were exempt from these customs.*

In fact, Silvia's baptism took place when she was just nine days old… and my parents were already planning to embark on a new adventure.

Life in Abbateggio had to come to an end, my mother wrote, *because there was no way papà could progress in his career. My cousin Vari visited us from Tanganyika. He spoke to us about Black Africa, and his stories were fascinating to a young man who was looking for a way out.*

My paternal grandfather was already well into his sixties, and my father wanted to be able to help support his two youngest brothers through medical school.

And so, on 30th March 1951, my father's twenty-seventh birthday, he and my twenty-two-year-old mother set off with a toddler and a two-month-old baby. Their parents lent them money for their passages, and to start them off. My father had no position lined up at the other end, but Vari assured them that there was a desperate need for doctors in Tanganyika. My mother and the children would stay with Vari, his wife Marta, and their ten-year-old daughter Rosaria, while my father travelled around the country looking for a job.

Various family members accompanied them in a minibus to Ciampino airport.

Just before they left, an aunt asked Enrico, 'Where are you off to?'

He shrugged his two-year-old shoulders and replied, '*Saccele-yè*,' which means 'How on earth should I know?' in the Abbateggio dialect.

This unknown destination turned out, in my father's words, to be *a leap into the light of an incredible experience, into a world light-years distant from ours, a world whose dimensions are so different from those in Europe, where one lives in another climate and another atmosphere.*

URAMBO, TANGANYIKA

March-May 1951

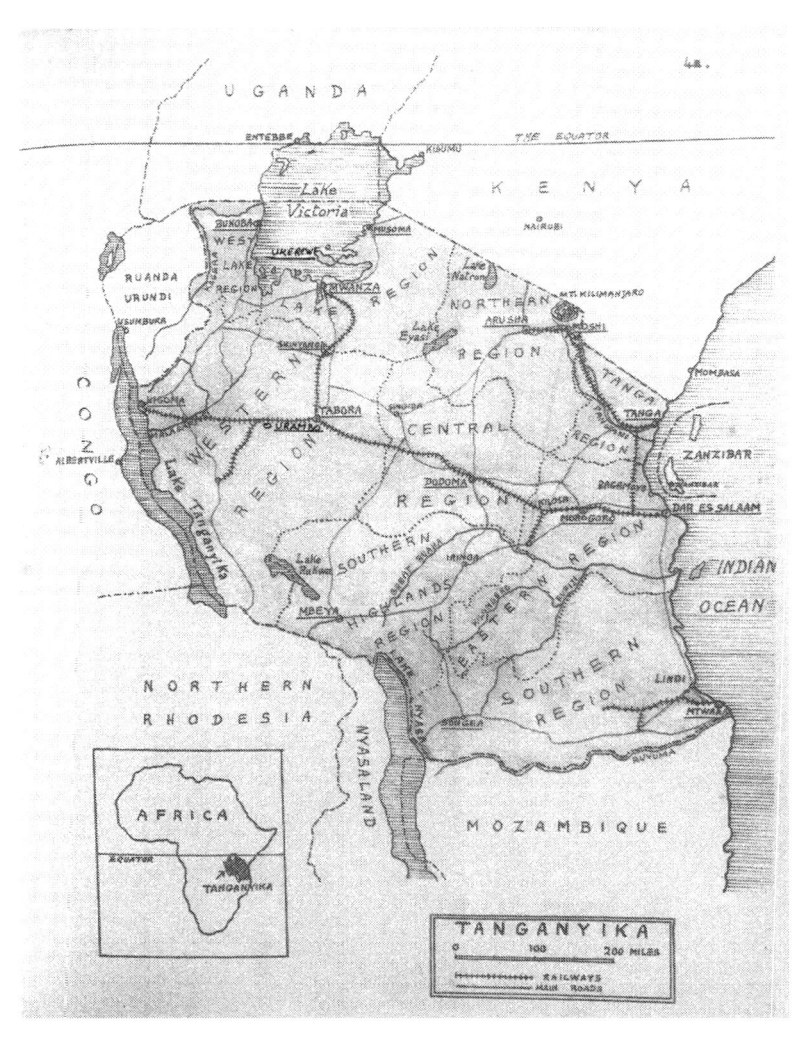

Map of Tanganyika drawn by my father

The Telegram

Tanzania came into being as a country in 1964, through the union of Tanganyika and Zanzibar. The country is three times the size of Italy, and lies just below the equator. The Indian Ocean laps its east coast, and the west is hemmed in by the long, deep Lakes Tanganyika and Malawi in the Rift Valley. To the northwest is Lake Victoria, which is almost as big as Ireland. Tanganyika was part of German East Africa from 1880 until the end of the First World War, after which it was placed under British administration as a League of Nations mandate.

My parents, brother, and sister flew to the capital, Dar es Salaam, via Cairo and Khartoum. From there a once-weekly plane took them to Urambo, a town 900 kilometres to the west, where Vari and his family were living. Having settled the family in, my father set off back to Dar es Salaam by train on his quest for work.

Vari had been a prisoner of war in Kenya, and was now employed by the Tanganyika Agricultural Corporation. He was an engineer, working on a project to clear the bush and build a dam to capture rainwater so the local people could grow crops. A number of English people worked on the project, alongside local employees.

I don't know how my mother would have managed without the support of the family, who were 'old Africa hands', while my father travelled around the country. The furthest from Italy she had ever been was a few kilometres across the Swiss border. And now here she was, 9,000 kilometres from home, in a place where everything was new to her: the language, the customs, the people.

She, and occasionally my father, wrote letters to her parents. Her cramped and rushed handwriting filled the flimsy blue airmail forms from top to bottom and often spilled onto the outside.

Urambo, 1st April 1951

We arrived on Friday. Vari, Marta and Rosaria gave us a warm welcome at the airport. Silvia was sick during the last leg, but she's happy now in her basket on the verandah, with the dog guarding her to ensure that not a single fly gets near her.

It's much more developed here than I expected: the Africans seem quite educated, the houses are lovely, the few shops sell everything you could need, from pins, toys, jam, and spaghetti to sewing machines.

Vari's home is delightful, and looks like it should belong to Snow White. The main house comprises a verandah, two bedrooms, a big living room, a bathroom and a storeroom. The kitchen, pantry and dining room are in another little house nearby. The African 'boy', Benedetto, lives in a third house with his wife and child.

Flowerbeds surround the main house; outside the kitchen are rows of tomatoes, parsley, onions, and garlic, and Benedetto grows his own vegetables outside his home.

As soon as Enrico saw Benedetto's son, Francis, he gave him a kiss.

Ugo will go to Dar es Salaam on Tuesday, to start looking for a job. Everyone says there's a desperate need for doctors here, but we need choose carefully.

The Telegram

Urambo, 18th April 1951

Since Ugo is not here, Vari is taking good care of us. He has decided that for Silvia's health, she needs to be taken out in the Land Rover, which is a sort of enormous Jeep. Today he took us for a ride, splashing through immense swamps. Vari, Marta, Enrico and I sat in the front, and behind were Silvia in her basket, and Rosaria.

It still feels like a dream to be in Africa. The rainy season is coming to an end: every day, after it has poured for a couple of hours, the sun comes out and dries everything instantly.

Today I received a letter from Ugo. All well in Dar es Salaam.

Urambo, 21st April 1951

Enrico talks about you all the time. Ugo has been offered several jobs, but he wants to think carefully before signing a contract, which will tie him down for two or three years.

We have never been separated for so long, but we are happy to make this sacrifice for our good and that of the children.

The climate is magnificent, between 18 and 24 degrees. And we're in the middle of a forest, so it's well ventilated. We often see monkeys nearby. Three days ago, a man went with three local 'boys' to hunt elephants, and shot one of the four they saw, a male, with tusks a metre and a half long.

On Tuesday I was taken with Silvia to a baby clinic, where there were several English mothers and babies. A nurse weighed the babies, and gave tips on feeding. Strangely, Silvia was the only breastfed baby. Here in Urambo, the English women wean their babies after two weeks.

Urambo, 5th May 1951

Today Enrico made his first sortie into society: the school held a party with dances and songs. Silvia came too, in her basket, dressed in a skirt, with a pink ribbon in her hair, but she stayed in the Land Rover beside us because the garden was too dusty.

I am obsessed with English: I hope Ugo will teach me a bit. I understand about fifty words out of fifty thousand. I'm going crazy with these blessed English people; each one speaks with a different accent.

Under Marta's guidance, I've taken up sewing. I am hopeless, but I love it all the same. It took me ages, but I managed to make a pair of dungarees for Enrico.

At the beginning of May, my father made a breakthrough in his job-hunting, and sent an update to his parents-in-law, in his clear, measured, and flowing handwriting.

Dar es Salaam, 5th May 1951

I will be going to Mwanza on the south coast of Lake Victoria to meet a bishop and discuss the terms of a contract with the Catholic Missions.

Everything is different here: people, customs, mentality; it takes a while to get used to it. I hope – in fact I am certain – that we're getting close to the end of this period. It's a useful life experience to be in a difficult situation, obliged to overcome discomfort and obstacles.

Soon afterwards, he sent a telegram to my mother:

> *ISOLA PARADISIACA TI ASPETTA*
> *[PARADISE ISLAND AWAITS YOU]*

The Bishop of Mwanza had spoken to my father about Ukerewe Island, on Lake Victoria. 'The Mission only has a small dispensary there,' he said, 'in a village called Kagunguli. We need to build a hospital. You could supervise the construction work, to your specifications, and remain there as a doctor. We would give you a three-year contract.' My father went with the bishop to visit the island. This offer of a secure job on a beautiful, fertile island, where there was work to be done, was exactly what he wanted. He accepted immediately and returned to Urambo to pick up the family.

UKEREWE

1951-1954

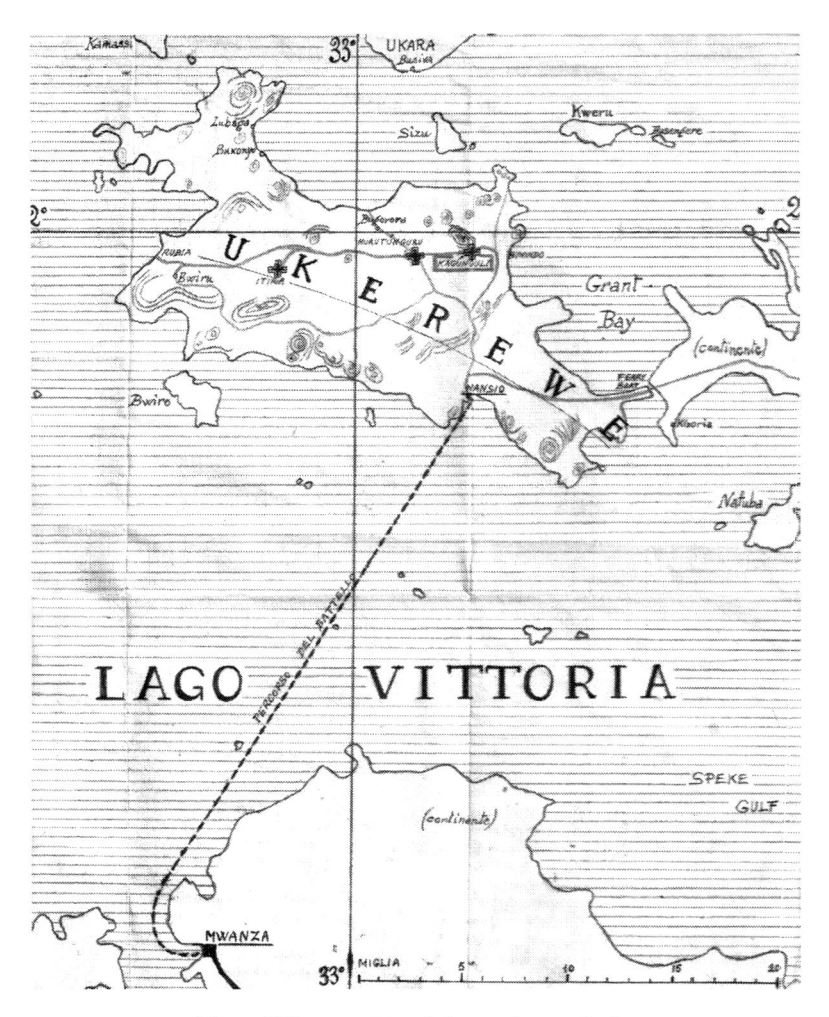

Map of Ukerewe Island drawn by my father

Paradise Island

On the way to Ukerewe, my father wrote to his parents-in-law.

Tabora, 26th May 1951

Here we are at last, travelling to our dream island on Lake Victoria. Isn't it romantic that we are going to live on a green island in the middle of an African lake, in a Catholic Mission surrounded by orange trees and palm trees?

We left Urambo at about half past ten this morning (Saturday), and at three this afternoon we arrived in this beautiful Tabora hotel.

Tomorrow evening we'll take the train to Mwanza, on the shore of Lake Victoria, where we will arrive on Monday morning. We have booked first class tickets so we will travel in comfort.

On Tuesday or Wednesday morning we'll take the boat to the island of UKEREWE (45 kilometres from Mwanza). We will send you news as soon as we are settled.

Here my mother takes over:

The children are sleeping, Enrico in his bed and Silvia in her basket. You can't think of Silvia without thinking of her basket because she's so happy in it: I only take her out to feed her.

Thank you for offering to send supplies. We need plates, pots and pans, crockery, medical books, bed and table linen.

Marta and Vari were so good to us: they generously and lovingly hosted us for two months without wanting anything in return. We will always be grateful to them.

Soon it will be dinnertime. They'll serve us the usual unseasoned concoctions, but we're getting used to them. On our island I will cook, my way. I can't wait to be there.

We bought a lovely English-style pram for Silvia, tall and wide with a big detachable parasol, green and beige.

*

Ukerewe Island is in the southeast corner of Lake Victoria. It's about the size of the Isle of Man, with an area of 530 km^2. A ferry links it to Tanzania's second-largest town, Mwanza. It takes almost four hours to make the crossing. Lake Victoria is only eighty metres deep and lies at an altitude of 1,100 metres.

A young Dutch priest met my parents when they arrived with Enrico and Silvia in Ukerewe's port, Nansio. He was over two metres tall, and his name was Father van der Wee.

'Did you bring everything?' he asked my mother. 'Everything you need to run a house… pots and pans, cutlery, crockery…'

The supplies from Italy would take a while to arrive. My mother had three heavy cases, mostly filled with nappies and clothes. So there in Nansio, she stocked up with what she thought would be necessary to start this new phase in her life.

As Father van der Wee drove the family on a dirt track fifteen kilometres north to Kagunguli, he explained that to start with, the family would have to live in temporary accommodation, while a house was built for them. Two domestic science rooms in the village school had been vacated for them.

There was no electricity, and no running water. They shared the rooms with hundreds of bats. *At night,* my mother reminisced, *in the flickering of the kerosene lamps, the bats looked like elephants against my mosquito net.* She had a bat phobia for the rest of her life. It was no reassurance when my father told her that bats breast-fed their babies just as she did.

*

My mother kept up her regular letters to her parents. Although my father's photographs may today look faded, the letters have lost none of their freshness.

Kagunguli, 1st June 1951

A rushed note. Ugo is at the hospital. I am at home sorting things out. The children are in the garden while Cecilia, the ayah, is washing their clothes. Vedastus, the boy, whose name I have trouble remembering, is tidying up. Both of them wear a big cross around their neck and are proud to work for the 'bwana mganga' *– the doctor.*

Yesterday we went to see the place where our 'villa' is being built. The plan looks lovely. There will be a living room, a dining room, our bedroom, the children's bedroom, a guest room, and a bathroom. The kitchen and pantry will be in a separate building, and beyond that will be the boys' quarters. We hope to be able to move there in two months.

Ugo's hospital is being built nearby.
The children are well.
I will write again when I have a moment of peace.

Kagunguli, 3rd June 1951

We are well. We have everything we need and are living like lords.

Ugo is doing the paperwork to pay you back what we owe you, but it may take some time.

This is heaven on earth, both economically and from the point of view of the climate, which is important for the children.

Out of Ukerewe's population of 70,000, twenty-nine are Europeans, eleven of whom live in Kagunguli: three priests, four nuns, and us.

Today the D.C. – the District Commissioner – who lives in Nansio, invited us to tea. He's married to an American and they have a daughter of Enrico's age. A lovely family.

Here we eat like the English: four times a day. At 7 we have breakfast: fried eggs, bread, butter, jam, fresh orange juice, tea with milk, a few biscuits, and fruit – usually pawpaw or bananas. We have lunch at midday, but we don't start with soup or pasta: just meat with two or three vegetables, fruit, and sometimes a milk pudding. English people never eat plain bread: they always have butter with it. We have adopted this custom. At 3.30 we have tea, which is like breakfast without the eggs. At 7 we have dinner with soup, meat, vegetables, and fruit.

Food is very cheap – cheaper than in Urambo because there are fewer Europeans here. The fish is excellent. The Mission gives us fruit and vegetables for free. I have never tasted such delicious milk. The nuns make cheese and butter from it.

The climate is wonderful. Although we are only 240 kilometres from the equator, it feels like spring all the time, perhaps because of the lake air, or perhaps because we are 1300 metres above sea level.

Silvia is an angel. Enrico adores her. Every now and then he goes to her basket and kisses and cuddles her. He says, 'Silvia, answer me: ooh,' and Silvia goes 'ooh' and they have long chats with their oohs and aahs.

The views are stunning: the lake is like an ocean.

Kagunguli, 14th June 1951

On Monday we invited the three Mission priests to dinner. One is from Alsace and two from Holland. Afterwards we had such fun playing cards, in a mixture of Latin, French, English, Swahili, Kikerewe, Italian and Dutch, so as to be able to understand each other.

One of the nuns is French-Canadian, two Dutch, and one German. Every now and then a nun comes to visit: the other day one taught me to ice cakes! Another is making me an evening dress. You might laugh, but here, the nuns are much more modern than in Italy, and they understand things!

Gifts are beginning to come in, just like 'il cumplimento' in Abbateggio: someone gave Ugo a hen, and the tribal chief came to greet us with a bunch of bananas.

I wasn't comfortable with the free produce from the Mission, so I made a deal: I give them three shillings a week for all the fruit and vegetables we need.

As soon as we are organised, Ugo will buy me a sewing machine, which will be useful for making clothes for the children and things for the house.

To answer your question, mamma, Ugo's contract provides for fifteen days' local leave every year, with travel paid to anywhere in Tanganyika, and three months' long leave at the end of the contract, with travel paid to anywhere in the world.

Kagunguli, 2nd July 1951

Yesterday, Sunday, we went to Rubia, the island's most beautiful beach, to have a picnic with the D.C.'s family. They came to pick us up in their car, and we loaded it with boxes, bags, pots, and even a tripod. We lit a fire and made ravioli with sauce, and coffee, and afterwards we washed the dishes in the lake. While Silvia lay gurgling in her basket, Enrico spent the whole day in the water, playing with the little English girl.

The other day a priest came from the mainland and went hunting in a truck with several guns. He was quite successful, and gave us a warthog he'd shot. We gave half of it to the Mission, and a lot to Cecilia and Vedastus. The meat is delicious, but we're sick of eating warthog!

Kagunguli, 2nd August 1951

Yesterday I baptised a baby who was born eight weeks premature, and I named her Vittoria Maria after you, mamma, and after Ugo's mother. I poured water on her head. If she survives, they will take her to the church for an official ceremony, but they will keep the name I gave her.

Kagunguli, 9th August 1951

You can't imagine how impatient we are to receive the boxes: if they haven't left yet, please could you add my kitchen scales? Before spending on superfluous things, we would like to clear our debt with you, and hope we will be able to send you something at the end of this month. We have been in Africa four months, but Ugo has only been working for two. We left Italy with 90 kilos of baggage, but have had to buy a lot of essentials: buckets, a baby bath, crockery, plates, pots and pans, bedding, and curtains. Mamma, could you send me my knitting magazines, and if you have one, a pattern book for children's clothes?

Kagunguli, 19th August 1951

A few days ago, an Indian man took us to see big game, in one of those amazingly long American cars. After hours of travelling, we ended up in the middle of an immense savanna where there were no roads. We saw eight giraffes, thousands of antelopes of various species, three ostriches, dozens of zebras and warthogs, but what was most interesting were animals that have a cow-like body, a dark brown hide, and a head a bit like a goat. They are called wilde-beest.

Kagunguli, 12th September 1951

Thank you for the good wishes for my name day. I've started teaching knitting to the Standard V girls once a week, and today they invited Mother Superior, the Headmistress, and Ugo to their classroom. Then they called for me, and when I arrived with the children, the girls all clapped their hands. They sang a song – I didn't understand a word – while a teacher beat the rhythm on a drum, and they gave me flowers, eggs, and straw tablemats. Enrico was stunned into silence, but Silvia laughed and clapped.

Kagunguli, 12th October 1951

I am writing from the garden. Silvia is sleeping, her hair braided into two plaits. Enrico is beside me, writing on his blackboard. You should hear how he speaks Swahili now, just like an African, with a perfect accent, aspirating all the 'h' sounds, and conjugating all the verbs correctly. He sings, counts, prays, talks, and thinks in Swahili.

I haven't yet told you about the Africans' names. The Christians choose saints' names for their babies, but the others have names like 'Motorcar', 'Bicycle', 'Born at Midday', 'Son of the Rain', 'Lightning', 'Cloud', or 'Tree.'

The people here are much cleaner than the people of Abbateggio. They have a complete wash every day, even if they are in hospital with a high fever. The children are impeccably clean and never smell: their mothers pour a bucket of water over them every day, even when they are newborns.

Kagunguli, 25th October 1951

Ugo was called to the hospital and I went to help him: a woman arrived who had been in labour for six days. She had a large tumour at the neck of her uterus, which was preventing the baby from coming out. Ugo managed the delivery, but it took him about half an hour to get the baby to cry.

Yesterday he operated on a man suffering from leprosy.

Kagunguli, 16th November 1951

Enrico has recovered well from measles, and his appetite is back to normal. Silvia is fine. Ugo says it's rare for children under two to catch measles and I hope that's true. She's happy to spend hours sitting in her high chair or on a mat with a raw carrot in her hand, which is great for me, as I'm busy preparing for the new house, filling cushions, making curtains and so on. A nun helps me, with her sewing machine. The house is almost finished and will be ready by the end of the month. The Standard Five girls from the school, who are between thirteen and fifteen (but who look about thirty), will help me clean before we move in.

School here is different from in Italy: they do academic subjects from 7.30 in the morning till midday, and from 2 to 5 they do housework: they sew, knit, clean the classrooms, do laundry, and if we need them, they work for me or the nuns.

Medical Matters

My father greatly admired Albert Schweitzer, the Lutheran theologian, philosopher and physician who spent much of his life working in West Africa, from 1913 onwards. There are some parallels between their work: forty years before my father, Schweitzer had built a missionary hospital in the town of Lambaréné, in Gabon, at a similar latitude to where my father was in East Africa. Schweitzer's hospital, like my father's, was in a remote area where there had previously been no doctor. And like Schweitzer, my father operated on thousands of patients, and devoted most of his career to working with disadvantaged communities.

Six months after his arrival in Ukerewe, the Roman newspaper *Il Messaggero* published a letter from my father.

Kagunguli, November 1951

> *For the last six months, I have been here, in the oldest of the three Catholic Missions of Ukerewe, a fertile island in the southeast corner of Lake Victoria. When, during a reconnoitring trip to Tanganyika, I reached Kagunguli, I immediately and enthusiastically decided I would return to work in the primitive*

little hospital of this Mission. Only here did I begin to discover the real Africa, with its immense needs, whereas before I had only heard about its immense resources.

There is no shortage of work: I am the only doctor on the island, which has a population of 70,000 people. This ratio may seem absurd in Europe; but here it isn't unusual. Until a few months ago, Ukerewe had never had a doctor.

So now, patients come to the little old hospital of Kagunguli with trust, even if all too often they arrive in such a state that the task of helping them seems hopeless. Despite the best will in the world, we sometimes feel incapable of doing anything for these poor patients who entrust themselves to our care. They almost always reach the hospital too late. Transport is hard to come by, and we have limited equipment.

Up to now I have always mentioned the word 'hospital': but this doesn't bear the faintest resemblance to a hospital as we know it in Europe. The main building is a small three-room house, which serves as an outpatients' department, a dispensary, and a pharmacy/rudimentary laboratory. Close by are half a dozen structures, most of them mud huts with thatched roofs, which are our 'wards': in total there is space for about twenty beds.

A nun works as an assistant to the patients, helped by a few local girls, and a male nurse carries out laboratory tests. The hospital, which has absolutely no modern facilities, contains a few pieces of old wooden furniture. In these conditions, operations can't be risked, apart from urgent cases or minor surgery: the wooden bed used for examinations serves as an operating table when it is needed.

What is happening in the little hospital at Kagunguli could be called pioneer work: but it must also be said that alongside the inevitable failures and disappointments, a huge number of satisfying achievements – especially in the field of obstetrics – give us the joy and courage to continue in this task of caring for the sick, while we *wait for the construction of our new modern hospital, which has been planned by our bishop, the Most Reverend Monsignor Blomjous.*

It will take time and money to realise this beautiful dream: but we have faith that one day, in the not too distant future, with our new, well-equipped hospital, we will be able to deal more efficiently with the needs of these poor people, who have never enjoyed any amenities, and whose lives are propped up only by a mysterious natural and spiritual energy.

*

Seven months after arriving on the island, the family was finally able to move out of the classrooms and into their own new home. Silvia's earliest memory is of her Kagunguli bedroom, painted green, my mother told us, 'because green is a soothing colour, good for children, and because when you opened the windows the green blended into the massive mango trees in the garden. So the walls were pale green and the curtains and bedspreads were pale green, covered with tiny designs of squirrels, dolls and baby elephants.'

Now the family had their own water supply, with two 1,000-gallon rainwater tanks in the garden. But this only collected enough water in the rainy season, and for many months of the year, my mother rationed the tank water, using it for drinking and cooking. Water for bathing, washing the clothes, and cleaning the house had to be brought from a dirty stream nearby, and boiled on a wood stove in the garden and left to settle as all the impurities drifted to the bottom. My mother planted pawpaw and banana trees in the garden, amongst the mango trees.

My father bought my mother a second-hand fridge. Meat was brought to the village from the port once a week, and now she no longer had to boil it all twice a day every day.

It must have been wonderful for my mother finally to be able to accommodate visitors.

Medical Matters

Kagunguli, 18th January 1952

At last, Vari, Marta and Rosaria are with us. It's such fun having them. They brought a beautiful gift: a huge brass Indian dish embossed by hand. Ugo will make legs for it, and we will use it as a coffee table.

Marta takes over the letter here.

Enrico is a lovely boy: he speaks Swahili perfectly and acts as an interpreter for everyone. Silvia is gorgeous: blonde and cheerful. Maria is well organised and communicates in several languages. Ugo is respected by everyone. The new house is beautiful: it has everything you could need: a vegetable garden, flowers, a good water supply, a luxurious bathroom, polished floors, curtains on all the windows, and a magnificent fridge. Rest assured that they are happy.

*

Finally, the long-awaited shipment arrived from Italy.

Kagunguli, 28th January 1952

The big news is that two days ago the famous boxes arrived. Very little was damaged. Two picture frames had come unstuck, but Ugo – doctor, surgeon, engineer, architect, blacksmith and carpenter – repaired them immediately. Thank you for everything. You can't imagine how useful the bed linen is. The house is even more beautiful now, and when the nuns popped in yesterday, they were amazed to see pictures on the wall, the clock, ornaments, and vases filled with flowers.

Kagunguli, 12th April 1952

This week's sensational news is that a lion swam over from the mainland and ate six cows. Our friend the D.C., with two guards and about a hundred men, managed to surround the lion and kill it. The Africans were all delighted: they danced all day and now the lion's skin is laid out at the D.C.'s office. This is the first time a lion has been seen on the island.

*

After a year on the island, the new hospital was ready. For my father, it was a dream come true. At last, he felt he had the resources to do his job properly. Soon he had qualified staff working under him: two State Registered Nurses, a medical assistant, and a midwife, helped out by several trainees. The Mission gave my father the use of a car – a Peugeot station wagon – to enable him to travel around the island to see patients: a step up from his Abbateggio mule days.

*

Kagunguli, 27th July 1952

This week Ugo performed his 12th cleft lip operation. Ugo is delighted, and so are the missionaries, because our hospital is building a reputation.

He has also learnt to do skin transplants. Tropical wounds can heal in two weeks with this method, whereas before, even wounds that were properly dressed and cared for could take up to six months to heal. He takes skin from a healthy part of the body and fixes it onto the wound. It's not real plastic surgery, but Ugo is proud of his success. He's learning all these new techniques from

Medical Matters

American books, which the bishop gave him. He sees about twenty-five patients a day, in addition to the forty who are in the hospital.

*

In August 1953, the family's local leave was interrupted by a medical emergency.

Kagunguli, 20th August 1953

As you can see, we're home already, though we weren't due back for another few days. We left Dar es Salaam on the 15th and arrived in Mwanza on the 17th, then went on to Bukumbi where Ugo was doing checkups on schoolchildren. Yesterday, some Indians came to fetch us because an Indian woman in Kagunguli was seriously ill with eclampsia. They found us by radioing the White Fathers in Mwanza. They managed to get the ferry to make a special crossing for us. We got to the hospital at midnight, which is why I am tired now.

The woman is in a bad way, and Ugo doesn't have much hope, though he is doing everything he can to save her.

We had a lovely holiday, but it would have been good not to have to end it so suddenly. When you are indispensable, you have to take the consequences.

The children are happy to be back: they prefer this backwater of Kagunguli to the city of Dar.

I can tell that the new baby is well, and strong, from the kicks I feel inside me.

24th August 1953

The Indian woman who was in agony picked up as soon as Ugo saw her. She's still quite unwell but she can talk, she's eating, and she can move every limb, whereas she had seemed completely paralysed when we arrived. Everyone says Ugo is incredible, but he says he didn't do anything special, and that the Good Lord decided to spare the mother so she could be with her ten children (the last of whom was born two days before our return).

The Ugly Baby

My goodness, that baby is ugly!
That's one ugly baby, is that.
Show me an uglier baby
And I'll eat the badge off my hat.

From *The Ugly Baby* by Jonathan Lamb

5th January 1954

ITALCABLE
I ARRIVED HAPPILY LAST NIGHT ALL WELL LOVE
FROM PAOLA

My father confirmed the news in a letter:

Kagunguli, 5th January 1954

Just a quick note to let you know about the happy event of Paola's birth last night at 10.25.

> *Everything went well, and she weighed in at 3 kilos. To me she looks rather ugly, but you can't really tell on the first day: she has a squashed nose, not much straight dark hair, and small eyes with few lashes. Apart from her nose, which I think she has taken from me, she's the image of Maria when she was small. But Maria became pretty, and Paola might too.*
>
> *Maria and the baby are fine. Enrico and Silvia are delighted. We will baptise Paola on 12th January, Silvia's third birthday.*

*

Enrico remembers a commotion on an evening a few months after my birth. 'You were sleeping in the room at the back,' he told me. 'A dead python was laid out along the front of the house. It was blotchy, green and brown, and enormous. It had swallowed a dog whole. Papà had killed it. I felt so proud! Imagine! My dad killed a python! We skinned it, and took the skin to Italy, and had shoes and bags made out of it.' The python was probably three or four metres long, but to his five-year-old eyes it stretched the whole length of the façade of our house.

The fact that my father killed a python surprises me: on his ninetieth birthday, in a filmed interview with my nephew, my father reminisced: 'The Missionaries once took me on a hunting expedition in the bush. I have never in my life held a weapon. A German priest, Father Junker, said to me, "See that wildebeest over there?" It was far in the distance. The priest fired one shot. We saw the animal fall. As we approached, he fired more shots.' Here my father paused and looked up at the camera. His eyes glistened. 'It was a female. She had a baby calf beside her. I will never forget how the calf looked up at me, her eyes pleading, "Why?"' He paused again. 'I could not answer.'

After three years on the island, my father's contract was coming to an end. Preparations had to be made to move on. My mother wrote to her parents from Mwanza.

The Ugly Baby

Mwanza, 9th June 1954

I'm in Mwanza with Paola, staying with Belgian friends, doing administration work regarding our departure from Ukerewe and trip to Italy for long leave. I have got our re-entry permits on our passports and have been to the vet to get a permit to take three python skins to Italy (one for you, one for Ugo's mother, and the third – the one Ugo killed – for me).

Enrico and Silvia are looking forward to the gifts I will bring them: Enrico asked for shoes with laces, like his father's; Silvia said any shoes would do as long as they are red.

Tomorrow Ugo will vaccinate all of us: I'm not looking forward to it as Paola will no doubt end up with a high fever. But it has to be done; they are strict here on international health regulations.

Kagunguli, 7th July 1954

We don't have any news about our next posting yet. The bishop sent Ugo a letter, saying how sad he is that Ugo is leaving, but that he understands our family reasons. He thanked him for the great work done at the hospital, and for his professional devotion.

Yesterday we went to see a film of the Queen's Coronation at the D.C.'s: the English ladies were moved to tears, I was bored, and Ugo, so as not to waste time, slept right through it.

Mwanza, 10th July 1954

Ugo will have told you the news. The important thing is that it's over and I am fine. My stitches are out and I can walk around the hospital. They have looked after me well: I didn't even notice the anaesthetic.

> *I'm sorry it had to happen now, and that Ugo has to look after the children, organise the move, and is worried about me.*
>
> *I think they took out both my ovaries with two cysts. I was a few weeks pregnant, but yesterday I miscarried. Now I can't have any more children, and that saddens me, because Ugo and I would have loved to have a little boy called Guido.*

My father wrote the last letter from Ukerewe.

> *Kagunguli, 12th July 1954*
>
> *Maria is well. She was operated on a week ago in Mwanza. You will understand that we didn't tell you anything before the operation. It would have been an unnecessary worry.*
>
> *There is an excellent surgeon in Mwanza, and they have a modern machine for anaesthetics.*
>
> *I am here alone with the three children. I have a lot to do, what with feeding Paola, looking after the hospital, and packing our things. Maria will be back today or tomorrow: she will be taken to the boat, and I will go to Nansio to fetch her in the car.*
>
> *We will see you very soon. We will fly from Mwanza to Entebbe in a local plane, spend the night in Entebbe, and leave the next morning in a Skymaster for Cairo, where we will spend another night. On Sunday morning, 25th July, we will leave for Rome.*

Years later, I asked my mother what it was like living in Ukerewe.

'I loved papá so much; I was happy.'

'Did you miss your parents?'

'Not really. They knew we were *bravi ragazzi* and that was enough for them. They didn't really know where we were, apart from "in Africa".'

'Did you get pleasure out of anything?'

'I was too busy. But in the evenings, we used to sit on the verandah and watch the sunset and the stars. After all, with no electricity, there wasn't much else to do after dark.'

ROME

July–November 1954

Long Leave

Imagine the changes in the three years since my parents had left Abruzzo. The village of Kagunguli had a new hospital, which functioned well, and the doctor's home had been built nearby. My father had encountered diseases he had never seen before. Through his experience, being the sole doctor for a huge population, he had become a specialist in every field: gynaecology, tropical diseases, ophthalmology, and surgery. I remember as a small child scrabbling in awe through a small box he kept, containing 'treasures' he'd removed from people's stomachs: my favourite was a small rusty arrowhead from those Ukerewe days.

'No, it wasn't meant for the man I operated on,' he reassured me. 'It was supposed to kill an animal someone needed for food. And don't worry, the man recovered well.'

The family had been exposed to Kikerewe, Swahili and English. My mother had undergone major surgery. And, almost miraculously, considering the cysts that had invaded her ovaries, she had a new baby.

In June 1954, we travelled to Rome by plane, a journey that took several days, and settled in with my mother's parents, who lived in the city centre. So much time, space and experience separated my parents from their previous Roman lives.

*

Did they feel different? How did all the relatives take to their stories of bats in the bedroom, pythons, and meat that had to be boiled twice a day? I imagine that it was exciting and exotic for everyone for a day or two, and then we gradually morphed into an Italian existence, being pampered by our maternal grandparents in their bourgeois apartment with rooms that were out of bounds for children and cold marble floors and priceless chandeliers, and shades tightly closed so the sunshine wouldn't spoil the heirloom furniture, and a spicy, smoky whiff wherever you went: my grandfather's cigars were scattered around in all the drawers to serve as mothballs.

My father returned to Tanganyika after a few weeks to organise the family's next move. During his three years on Ukerewe Island, word of his success had spread, and he had been offered a job with the government, as District Medical Officer in the town of Musoma, on the eastern shore of Lake Victoria. The salary was double what he had earned with the Mission. He would be responsible for a well-established hospital and twelve district dispensaries. This promised the young family stability for the future. Musoma was a real town, with streets, shops, and an established, if small, European community. The island had been an adventurous and exciting start, but offered no long-term opportunities. The move to Musoma was to be the first of many upward steps.

Before he left Rome, my father, assisted by his dentist brother Ennio, removed Enrico's tonsils, probably in his parents' kitchen. 'It was pretty sore,' Enrico recalls. 'I can still remember the smell of the ether they used to anaesthetise me.'

My mother remained in Rome with us children, waiting for the official paperwork to arrive from the British Government to allow us to travel. Meanwhile, she stocked up on what she would need in Musoma: clothes and shoes for everyone, seeds for flowers and vegetables, new cutlery. Occasionally she went to the cinema with her brothers. She made frequent trips with us across Rome to visit my father's chaotically large family. Enrico enthusiastically joined his cousin Gianni at nursery.

I imagine my mother borrowed winter clothes for us all as summer turned to autumn and autumn to winter. In a letter to my father, she wrote:

It's so strange to think of you in short sleeves. Here it's freezing, but thank goodness the radiators are on. They say the cold is exceptional. Imagine, in Florence they recorded −4°: this is the coldest it's been in November since 1813 when records began.

Back in Tanganyika, my father bought his first car, a Vauxhall Wyvern. It was transported by train from Dar es Salaam to Mwanza, where he picked it up and drove it the two hundred kilometres east and north around the lake to Musoma, along with most of the luggage that had arrived from Ukerewe and was being stored at the Mission in Mwanza. Their original three cases had now become four, and in addition they had two chests and a hatbox containing crockery.

I arrived in Musoma yesterday at 5 p.m., my father wrote to my mother, *after a magnificent four-and-a-half-hour drive. I say magnificent because it was cool, and because our car runs superbly. I'm not talking about speed, because I'm still running it in and have to keep it to 35–40 m.p.h.; I mean that the engine runs as smoothly as oil. The road was in good condition, especially the last eighty kilometres from the Ukerewe turnoff to Musoma…*

The hospital is well organised, and incomparably better than the one in Mwanza.

My first impression is that Musoma is a beautiful place, and friendly too: I'm sure we'll be happy here.

Musoma has a club, a tennis court, a cinema, and many shops.

And on 11th December 1954, three weeks before my first birthday, my mother and we three children left Rome on Caspar Airways Flight BA 161, bound, via Entebbe, for our new home in Musoma.

MUSOMA

1954-1957

Musoma Memories

The early stories have been told over and over again. I remember the five of us sitting around the old wooden table in my parents' flat in Rome, where they lived for the three decades after their retirement, and where our frequent visits from our homes scattered around the world would sometimes coincide. That table, along with six matching chairs, had been found in pieces, some half-buried, some strewn around the garden of their last pre-retirement home, on Kinondoni Road in Dar es Salaam. That was the African home that lasted the longest: almost twenty years. My parents gathered up the dirt-encrusted planks, legs, seats, and backs, and my father pieced them all together, and sanded and varnished them. That table, which went with them to Rome after two decades in our open verandah dining room, was the hub of our conversations, which invariably turned to those African days.

Around that table photos and memories merged. I see the five of us poring over an album, each photo neatly captioned.

*

Minds flashed back; stories spilled.
'Oh look! Our first house in Musoma!' Silvia says. 'It was built

on a *kopje*. The kitchen was separate from the house and a gigantic sloping rock connected the two.'

And my father turns to his meticulously drawn house plan.

Silvia continues, 'I remember one day we were playing outside in front of the house, and a woman came running up screaming and covered in blood – I think her husband had taken a *panga* to her. We were quickly shooed into the house while papà took care of her.'

My mother interrupts. 'The road that led from that house to the hospital was named Fornari Avenue after we left, in honour of the work papà did.'

And more maps and plans are produced. And Silvia continues her story.

'Little mushrooms grew under the acacia trees in front of the house. I spent hours looking for fairies in them. I must have been four or five. Musoma was where my fascination for insects began. I discovered ant lions that made funnels in the sand, and lay hidden at the bottom. Ants slid down the slippery sides and the ant lions shot out their long pincers to grab and eat them.

'Once I was climbing over a fallen tree between the next-door neighbours and us, and a chameleon crawled into my skirt – I was terrified.

'We had a *shamba* by the path between the house and the lake, where we grew vegetables, and I can remember one night a hippo trampled all over it and in the morning we saw his great big footprints there.'

'Oh yes,' my mother says. 'The house was by the lake. You used to swim right there, at the bottom of the garden, but then people started seeing hippos and crocs, so I'd take you to a fenced-off part of the lake at the club.'

Years later, the hippo anecdote was adapted by an enthusiastic and creative Italian journalist. 'What are your most treasured memories of Lake Victoria?' he asked my father, and claimed that my father replied, 'The hippos who came and wrecked our vegetable patch at night, and who chased my children as they swam in the lake.'

My mother remembered that Enrico measured my father's prestige by the ambulances, truck, and Land Rovers owned by the hospital… and of course, by our very own Vauxhall. I measured it by the letters after his name, which I learned to recognise, representing his title: D.M.O. — District Medical Officer.

The Dress often featured in our round-the-table conversations in Rome.

*

'Remember mamma's black dress?' says Silvia.

My mother's eyes light up. 'Oh, I loved that dress!'

And my father, as precise as ever, goes into the details, smiling faintly. 'I won a prize for doing well in a Swahili exam. Four hundred shillings. I spent it on buying two evening dresses for mamma. I bought them in Dar es Salaam.'

And the pages of the photo album are turned.

The photos show the dresses, calf-length, and flared from my mother's tiny waist. One is white, covered with layers of netting, with fine beaded straps. The other is black, with an off-the-shoulder neckline, embossed with red cherries. My mother wears a delicate string of pearls. In one photo she wears black high-heeled shoes, in the other, white ones. She oozes elegance. The white dress means nothing to me. It has no place in my memory. But I can still feel the cool, stiff taffeta of the black one: I can catch the faint mothball whiff wafting from it; I can feel my three-year-old heart swell with pride as I look up at my mother. This is what makes the difference between stories and real memories.

'Ah look, there we are on the way to Nairobi!' my father says, showing a photo in which our Vauxhall is stopped on the road in the middle of the savannah. Silvia is leaning out of a window and I am in the driver's seat. 'That's when we took Enrico to school for the first time.' My mother stiffens.

When the family travelled by car to take Enrico, aged seven, to St Mary's in Nairobi, my mother's parents vented their horror in a letter to her. She was adamant in her defence, and wrote to them:

Enrico, like all children, needs education. I schooled him for as long as I could. It's difficult to teach your own children, and I had to do it in a language that I am only learning myself. I have taught him to write, read and do some arithmetic, in my own improvised way. We looked hard for a good school, and St Mary's is magnificent.

It was with a heavy heart that we left him at the school. He was a little disoriented, but not unhappy. I was in floods of tears for having left him when I received your letter expressing your shock at our behaviour towards a poor innocent child, reprimanding me for being a negligent mother. I visited him two weeks later: he was happy, suntanned, chatting about all his adventures. He likes school, he likes the food, he likes sports...

After that first time, Enrico travelled alone, by plane. He is still amazed when he thinks back to the Musoma airstrip. 'Imagine! Small planes with propellers landed straight onto the grass!'

'How did you do at school when you arrived?' I asked him recently.

'Always in the top three in every subject. Except perhaps history.'

'And how did you feel, going to school so young?'

'Fine.'

My first friend was our Dalmatian, Fido. The memory of his cold wet nose and slobbery tongue is real... and I still feel the tears and sadness that engulfed me when Fido was sent to another home because my mother thought it was unhygienic for me to share my biscuits with him.

In my mind, I see our sitting room, with its Public Works

Department furniture that every government official's house contained. On a small table in the corner stands a radio. I see us sitting in the adjoining dining room, me fiddling around with the spoon in my soup. It's evening, and a Tilley lamp flickers on the table, casting shadows on the wall. A few flying ants and moths cluster around it. The acrid smell of paraffin fills the air. Enrico disappears for a few seconds, and a crackly voice booms through in Swahili. Enrico reappears giggling, saying, 'That's Malingumu… he's going to come and get you, Titch, if you don't eat your food!' Malingumu is the scariest bogeyman in the universe. And my parents send Enrico back to switch off the radio.

In that sitting room is a beige carpet. I have a bird's eye view of myself wearing a white cotton dress with smocking around the neck. I am skipping around the carpet, trying to keep within its borders. My fair doubled-up plaits bounce as I skip. My father is sitting in a wooden armchair, strumming his mandolin. He's playing *Treccine d'Oro*, a traditional Neapolitan tarantella. Is this a memory of a photo, of a story told a hundred times at the old wooden table, or is it a real memory? Does it matter? What I can swear to is the genuineness of that soaring feeling in my heart, which says: *This is my song and my father is playing it for me.*

BROMLEY, KENT

1957-1958

Smog

In summer 1957 we left what had been my home on Lake Victoria for most of my life, and travelled to Italy by ship, through the Suez Canal, on the *Lloyd Triestino Europa*.

A local newspaper published this article:

Popular Doctor Leaves Musoma
Almost all the Musoma town officials attended the sundowner given by the Musoma Government Hospital staff in honour of Dr. and Mrs. Fornari, who are shortly going on leave to Italy.

Mr. F.W. Weeks, Musoma District Commissioner, in paying tribute to the doctor's services in East Lake, said that most people in Musoma, including himself, had had the benefit of the doctor's patient, selfless, untiring and skilled services.

Other speeches paying tribute to the doctor's work were made by the Chief Clerk and Mr. M.O. Ngonga, Medical Assistant, on behalf of the medical staff, who expressed regret at losing their leader, who was, in addition, a psychologist and a philosopher; and Mr. M.G. Kayuza, headmaster of Musoma Middle School, on behalf of the education department, who expressed thanks for the doctor's keen interest in the welfare of school children.

> *In reply, Dr. Fornari thanked those who had come to the sundowner and the medical staff who had organised it. He hoped they would show the same love and loyalty to his successor as they had shown to him.*

Sundowner. I remember loving that word. I can imagine my father, a reserved teetotaller, uncomfortably sipping a Coke as people milled around from group to group, then, with his ever-quiet voice, making his farewell speech.

My memories of the trip by ship up the east coast of Africa and through the Suez Canal are few and sketchy: a swimming pool on deck that seemed as big as a lake, a terrifying King Neptune emerging from the depths of the ocean (in my mind, anyway) with his crown and his trident; Silvia falling into the pool – or perhaps King Neptune threw her in; not being able to disembark in Egypt because Silvia and I were violently ill; the smoky smell of leather when my father and Enrico came back from a trip ashore with a pouffe they had bought. Enrico remembers that they climbed on the walls of the pyramids and rode a camel.

We holidayed in Italy, once more catching up with the family. Several cousins had been born in the three years since our last visit. I was excited to learn that my father's sister Teta had a real live baby, her third child, growing in her big tummy.

In October 1957, we travelled via Calais and Dover to Bromley, in Kent, where my father, sponsored by the British Government in Tanganyika, embarked on a six-month course for a Diploma in Tropical Medicine and Hygiene at the University of London. Mary Hancock, an English teacher friend in Tanganyika, had found us a house to live in: the doctor who owned it was away studying in the U.S. Mary lent us a car she had in England: it looked like a London cab, and was a 1938 Lanchester 11. Silvia and Enrico remember the excitement of my father cranking it up every morning before he left for university.

Bromley was cold and dark. I learnt the word *smog*, and loved that it was made up of two words: *smoke* and *fog*. In my memory, a thick wet blanket covered the sky, holding in the smog, for the whole time we were there. My mother often reminisced that we had to fumble our way along the streets, feeling the walls and counting the houses, when we did the school walk. She didn't have time to plait my hair before we left the house in the mornings, so she would do it when we returned home, when she could get me to sit still for the time it took. My father, always a neat man, didn't like me looking so unkempt, so the plaits were chopped off.

I recall helping my mother bring in the washing from the outside line, and finding it frozen and hard. The 'smoke' that came out of my mouth when I breathed fascinated me.

This is where I learnt to read, I don't know how – probably just by watching Enrico and Silvia. My mother used to tell the story of us walking down a London street one day. I looked at a sign and said, 'That says "Bookshop".'

'How do you know?' she asked.

I replied, 'Because it's B-O-O-K for "book" and "S-H-O-P" for "shop".' It might have been simpler to deduce that it said 'Bookshop' because there were books in the window.

I learnt to write, and in January 1958, when I was just four, I crafted a letter in Italian to my paternal grandfather, Giulio. Below my illegible, misspelt, albeit well-intentioned scrawl, my father wrote a neat transcription: *Dear and beautiful Nonno Giulio, tell me what Zia Teta's new baby is called. Later I will come.*

The London period must have been difficult for my mother. She had spent her nine years of married life so far in a God-forsaken outpost in Abruzzo, a remote lake island, and a small dusty town on the equator. This was her first adult experience of a big city. She was in a strange country, and didn't know a soul. Her days were spent looking after three small children and a home that wasn't her own.

Meanwhile, my father was relishing his university experience. He followed his classes conscientiously, and we still have his handwritten notes from that time, together with detailed drawings of insects, worms and micro-organisms. He was absorbed by the mystery of the life cycle of these creatures. You could see the excitement on his face as he shared what he learnt with us, drawing neat diagrams as he spoke: 'When a mosquito bites you in the tropics, you may get malaria. Only the female carries the malaria parasite. First she has to find a suitable mate. Then she needs to find food, so her eggs can grow. That food is human blood.'

He told us about fleas. Like the mosquito, the plague-transmitting flea – again, always female – has to undergo hardships. At the time of biting, in order to get blood – like the mosquito, to prepare her eggs – she has to suck up the blood after vomiting masses of the plague bacilli that fill her salivary glands.

It was in London, through tests at the university, that my father, Enrico, and Silvia were diagnosed with bilharzia, which is a disease affecting the urinary or intestinal tract. It is caused by a worm, which has a double life cycle, one in snails, and one in the human being. It is common around Lake Victoria, in places where the water is stagnant. This is how it works: a child urinates into the lake. The urine contains eggs of the worm, which hatch in the lake. The larvae from the egg crawl into a particular type of snail. After a few weeks, the snail excretes adult larvae of worms, which penetrate the skin of humans. Eventually they settle in the blood system, where they grow and reproduce, and the cycle starts again.

My father always smiled as he told us these stories. 'The male worm is smaller than the female. The couple live monogamously in their less than heavenly surroundings. At this stage they are big enough to be visible to the naked eye. As a result of their love, thousands of eggs, provided with an appropriate spike, make their way through the wall of the blood vessel and bladder or rectum, and are thereby excreted. And so the wheel turns again.' He added wryly, 'What an intelligent design.'

The bilharzia contracted by the members of my family was 'subclinical' which means not serious. They must have caught it on Ukerewe Island, where my mother and I didn't swim, before my father had learnt about the disease. It gave them no symptoms, and soon cleared up with medication. In its full-blown form, there is continuous loss of blood in the urine or faeces, and the sufferers become weak and anaemic.

My father shared the anguish of all these tiny creatures, which had to suffer for their species to survive. He always told us that pairs of fleas, mosquitoes, and microscopic worms must have sailed side by side with elephants and cows in Noah's Ark. Perhaps this period of study contributed to his loss of faith.

I remember the day my father came home from university and told us it was time to move back to Tanganyika.

'We're going to Kigoma, on Lake Tanganyika,' he said. He explained that it was a long, narrow lake, not a round one like Lake Victoria. 'And it's so deep, that bilharzia worms can't live there. So we can swim safely.'

And so to a new home, and new adventures.

LETTERS FROM BROMLEY

Leap Into the Light

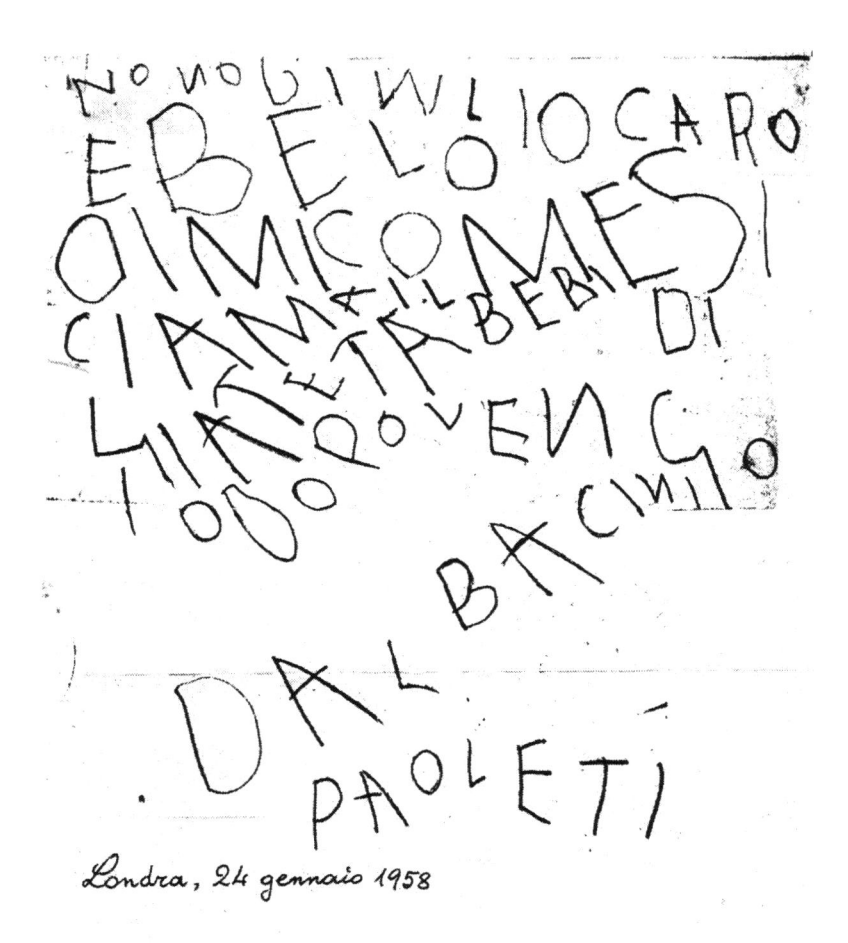

Londra, 24 gennaio 1958

Nono Giwlio caro e belo dimi come si ciama il bebi di zia Teta io dopo vengo bacini dal Paoleti

(letterina scritta da Londra da Paola di 4 anni al nonno Giulio).

My letter to our paternal grandfather, 1958
(Translation on page 67)

Letters from Bromley

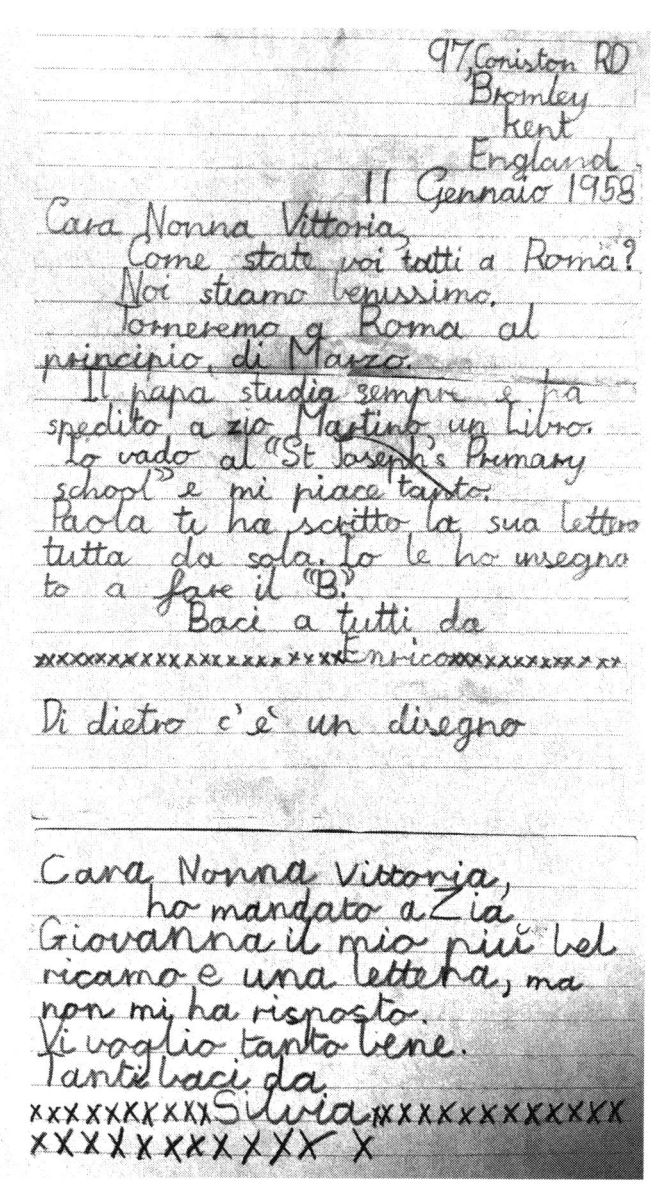

> 97, Coniston RD
> Bromley
> Kent
> England.
> 11 Gennaio 1958
>
> Cara Nonna Vittoria,
> Come state voi tutti a Roma?
> Noi stiamo benissimo.
> Torneremo a Roma al principio di Marzo.
> Il papà studia sempre e ha spedito a zio Martino un libro.
> Io vado al "St Joseph's Primary school" e mi piace tanto.
> Paola ti ha scritto la sua lettera tutta da sola. Io le ho insegnato a fare il "B."
> Baci a tutti da
> xxxxxxxxxxxxxxxxxxxxEnricoxxxxxxxxxxxx
>
> Di dietro c'è un disegno
>
> ---
>
> Cara Nonna Vittoria,
> ho mandato a Zia Giovanna il mio più bel ricamo e una lettera, ma non mi ha risposto.
> Ti voglio tanto bene.
> Tanti baci da
> xxxxxxxxxxSilviaxxxxxxxxxxx
> xxxxxxxxxxx x

Silvia and Enrico's letter to our maternal grandmother, 1958

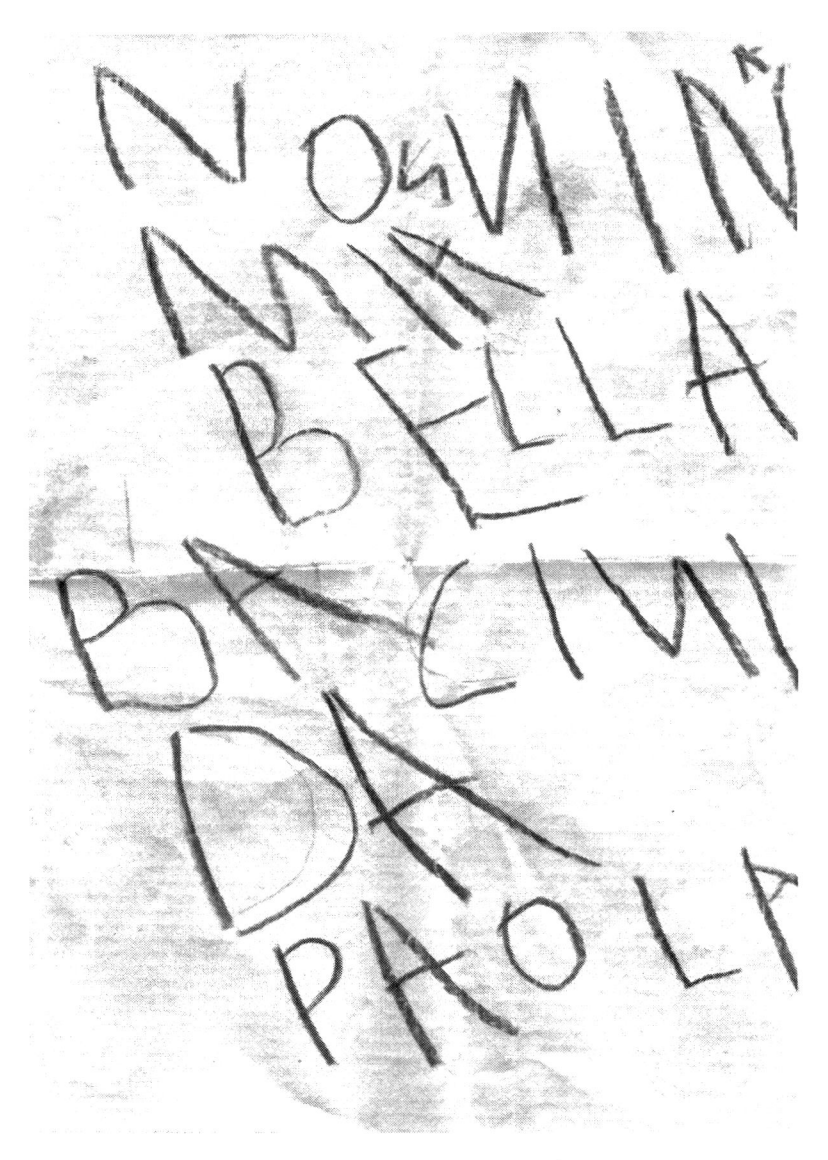

Leap Into the Light

My letter to our maternal grandmother, 1958

Translation of Enrico's letter:

Dear Nonna Vittoria,
How are you all in Rome?
We are very well.
We will return to Rome at the beginning of March.
Papá studies all the time and he sent zio Martino [my mother's brother] *a book. I go to "St Joseph's Primary School" and I like it very much.*
Paola wrote her letter all by herself. I taught her how to write the "B".
Kisses to everyone,
XXXXXEnricoXXXXX

At the back there's a drawing

Translation of Silvia's letter:

Dear Nonna Vittoria,
I sent zia Giovanna [my grandmother's sister] *my most beautiful embroidery, but she didn't reply.*
I love you very much.
Lots of kisses from
XXXXXSilviaXXXXX

Translation of my letter:

My beautiful nonnina kisses from Paola

KIGOMA

1958-1961

The Kaiserhof

The town of Kigoma is not far from the Burundi border, on the shore of Lake Tanganyika, the second-deepest lake in the world, which snakes for seven hundred kilometres down the western branch of the Great Rift Valley. From Kigoma, you can see the high escarpment of the Congo hills to the west. At its broadest point, the lake is only seventy-four kilometres wide.

The Central Railway Line crosses the entire country from Dar es Salaam on the east coast to Kigoma, a distance of over 1,200 kilometres. In our day it took fifty-eight hours to travel the length of the line: today it takes forty. The main line, built by the Germans, followed the old Arab slave route, and was completed just before the First World War. Another branch, completed by the British in 1928, branches north from Tabora to Mwanza on Lake Victoria.

Kaiser Wilhelm II, the last German emperor, was supposed to visit German East Africa and open the main line, but the outbreak of the war prevented him from travelling to this outpost of his empire. He never got to stay in either of the two identical buildings, both called the Kaiserhof – the Kaiser's House – which had been constructed especially for him, one in Kigoma, and one in Tabora.

When Tanganyika came under British administration after the war, the Kigoma Kaiserhof became the residence of the District Commissioner. As befitting an emperor, it was a magnificent building set on a hill overlooking the lake, with broad steps sweeping down from the verandah to the extensive grounds below. A more modest building, the Kaiserhof Annexe, designed to accommodate the Kaiser's staff, was assigned to the District Medical Officer.

We arrived in Kigoma in April 1958, after our six-month stint in London, and moved into the annexe. It had a square turret at each end of a long arched verandah: to us it was a palace.

The District Commissioner at the time was Walter Warrell-Bowring. I remember him as being tall, and wearing a cravat. A path linked our two homes, and we shared what seemed to me to be an infinite garden – a whole universe – to explore, with rocks and mango trees and prickly pear plants and elephant grass. Giant pods dangled and rattled from a colossal kapok tree, and when they ripened and opened my mother would sneeze and her eyes would water for days on end.

Jenny, the Warrell-Bowrings' eldest daughter, who was a year or two younger than I, was my first friend. While Enrico and Silvia were away at boarding school, Jenny and I were homeschooled by our mums.

I remember Mary Warrell-Bowring as a friendly, bubbly person. She and my mother were good friends. After my lessons, Jenny and I ran wild. Jenny's family had a dachshund, and ours a boxer cross, whose mother a leopard had mauled. My father had sewn up the badly injured dog and saved her life, and the owners gave us one of her pups, Rupert, as a thank you present.

One of my first memories of Kigoma is of walking through rustling long grass with Mary Warrell-Bowring, who was pregnant with her third child. I must have been five.

'What will you call your new baby?' I asked her.

'Victoria Anne or Stephanie June,' she replied. I remember wondering how she was so sure she would have a girl, and thinking how pretty those names were. But it also puzzled me that she should have chosen those particular combinations. Why not Victoria June or Stephanie Anne?

'What would you like to be when you grow up?' Mary asked me.

'A gynaecologist,' I said, with no hesitation.

'A gynaecologist? Why?'

'Because they look after babies, and I love babies.'

So Mary explained to me that gynaecologists looked after mothers who were going to have babies, and paediatricians looked after babies.

My father, who delivered around 5,000 babies over his career, used to take me to the wards at the hospital to see the new-borns. I guess this is where I learnt the word *gynaecologist*. Often the mothers asked me to name their babies. At the time, my favourite names were Christina and Crispino. I wonder whether any sixty-five-year-old Christinas and Crispinos are still living in Kigoma today.

We and the Warrell-Bowrings were great friends with José and Colin Lamb. Colin, Walter and my father all spoke fluent Swahili. Colin was the Inspector of Police working in the Special Branch, and José worked as Walter's P.A.. Colin and José were married in 1960 in Kigoma, by Walter. Their reception, held in the Kaiserhof verandah, was a magnificent affair. I am still in touch with José and recently we chatted about her wedding.

'I met Colin in Nairobi,' she said. 'I'd known him for five weeks when we got married, and I'd only seen him for a couple of days. All twenty-seven of the European community in Kigoma were there at the wedding. Your mother and Mary and the other ladies all made hats for the occasion. Imagine! Hats!'

José's memory is sharp, and she loves to talk about the Africa days. 'Do you remember the *dagaa*?' she asked me.

Dagaa are tiny fish, similar to whitebait. I will never forget their smell, their taste, their texture…

'We'd sit in the verandah and watch the fishermen after sunset,' José reminisced. 'They went out on moonless nights in their canoes with lamps. A sparkling necklace of lights lit up the bay. The lights would attract the fish.' As José spoke, the lights twinkled in my mind and in her eyes.

The fishermen would bring in their bursting nets and when the sun rose, the lakeshore would glisten with thousands of fish left out to dry. We would eat heaps of them whole: crunchy and salty with an added tangy squeeze of lime… simply exquisite. Forty years later I was back in Kigoma, and asked in my hotel if I could have *dagaa* for dinner. The manager was surprised, this being a 'popular' dish, but he sent out for some. I was in heaven.

Some years after our family left Kigoma my father delivered José and Colin's second daughter in Mwanza, and a few years after that helped bring Walter and Mary's son into the world in Dar es Salaam. My parents remained in touch with both families throughout their retirement, and I was delighted to recently re-establish contact with Jenny, who had been my first playmate… and I hers. Perhaps we will meet again.

Trains, Boats, and a Ferry

In 1958, when Silvia was seven, she started school at Loreto Convent Msongari in Nairobi, next door to Enrico's school, St. Mary's. There were no 'good' schools in Kigoma, and Europeans back then either sent their children to boarding school in the U.K., or in Nairobi. Our two Catholic schools were considered among the best in East Africa.

The first time Silvia went to school, we all accompanied her to Nairobi in our Volkswagen Beetle, which had a space behind the rear seat for luggage. We called that space 'the back of the back', and I felt hugely privileged to be allowed to sit there. The car's indicators were little orange bars that popped out between the front and back doors – a step up from hand signals.

My father often recited the itinerary of this epic trip to us like a litany: Kigoma–Kibondo–Mwanza–Musoma–Tarime–Kisii–Kericho–Naivasha–Nairobi–Arusha–Dodoma–Iringa–Mbeya–Mpulungu (on the south coast of Lake Tanganyika) by car – a distance of about 3,000 kilometres, and then our car was put on a boat, and we sailed the final 450 kilometres up the lake. It was a huge clockwise circle.

I remember us stopping to let an elephant cross the road at

one point. The colossal bull, his tusks held high, paused in the middle of the road, turned his head towards us, stared, and sauntered off.

The round trip took us a couple of weeks. We stayed in government 'rest houses' on the way, and the canvas basins and camp beds were, to me, the height of luxury.

When my father told us there would be ferries to take us across rivers along the way, I understood *fairies*. I was thrilled by this, and was deeply disappointed when I discovered the truth. The ferry was a rickety platform of wood, which floated between two parallel ropes strung across the river. You drove your car onto the platform, and four men sitting on either side would pull the ropes, hauling the car and passengers across.

After that first trip, Silvia and Enrico made the school trip together by train and steamer. The distance between Kigoma and Nairobi is about 900 kilometres as the crow flies, but their journey must have been double that distance. They came home only for Christmas, Easter and summer holidays.

They set off from Kigoma Station, a majestic structure built by the Germans before the First World War, in much the same style as the Kaiserhof. The train chugged off to the east, through groves of mango trees that had been planted along the old slave route. 'Before leaving, we prepared water bombs, by soaking crunched up paper balls in water,' Enrico remembers. 'We'd throw them at the people on the platform who were watching the train leave. The train took us to Tabora where we spent a night at a mission run by priests. The next day we took another train north from Tabora to Mwanza, stopping at several stations along the way. In Mwanza we walked to the port, and boarded a steamer, the *Victoria*, which sailed around the lake to Kisumu in Kenya. If the boat went anti-clockwise, via Musoma, we spent just one night on the boat, but if it happened to be going clockwise, the trip took two nights, via Bukoba and Kampala. We'd dock at Kisumu in the early morning, walk to another mission where the priests would give us lunch, then we'd take the overnight train through the Rift Valley to Nairobi.'

It took them between five and six days. Kigoma was at 'the end of the line', and as the journey progressed, more 'Saints boys' and 'Convent girls' would join them.

On the final leg of the journey, between Kisumu and Nairobi, 'chicken' was played: the most daring of the Saints boys would hop off the train at stations and hang about on the platform till the last minute, when the train started pulling out, to give chase and leap on again. The longer you waited, the more kudos you earned. On at least one occasion, a boy was left stranded at a cold station on the Rift Valley escarpment. I'm not sure if that made him more or less of a hero. This is how Silvia remembers the school journey:

'I never got to celebrate my birthday: school started in the second week of January and my birthday was either on arrival date, departure date or during the trip. I loved the train. At mealtimes a man used to come up and down the carriages announcing food with a xylophone. I remember the sheets were white and starched as stiff as boards and we had scratchy grey army blankets. I don't think anyone looked after us on the way – if someone did, they did a pretty lousy job because the kids used to buy cigarettes. You had to smoke to have any sort of prestige – I think the reason I have never smoked is because of the trauma of being given a *ten centi* when I was about eight. Cigs were passed around and I quickly learned that when it was my turn, if I blew instead of inhaling, the end would light up so I would look as cool as the others. People saw us off on the train and steamer and the nuns and priests picked us up at the station in Nairobi. On the trip, the 'big girls' and 'big boys', who must have been all of fourteen or fifteen, were in charge of the little ones. Sometimes there weren't enough cabins on the steamer so some of us (never me) could sleep on deck – usually it was the boys who did… and I was filled with envy. In Kisumu or Mwanza (the start of the boat trip one way or the other) there was a man on the dock who used to play a local trumpet and his cheeks would inflate like balloons. People would throw him money from the steamer but if we threw one-cent bits he'd throw them back at us.'

When I think of those trips to school, I imagine a giant multi-legged spider, each leg being a route carrying children from far-flung corners of East Africa to the body, Nairobi, in the centre.

And every child had a unique experience. Recently, Jerry Bary, a good schoolfriend of Enrico's, told me about his. He and his brother Eddy used to travel to Nairobi from Tanga, north of Dar es Salaam on the Indian Ocean, a trip that took two days and two nights. 'I hated travelling to Nairobi,' he told me, 'but I loved coming back!' Jerry explained that before he and his brother left, his father would give him cash to cover the term's books, outings, and pocket money, for both boys. 'I would stuff the wad in my underpants,' Jerry recounted, 'because I was dead scared that I would lose it, or that it would be stolen… what a relief, once at school, to hand it over to the Dean of Discipline! So while all the other children on the train had great fun, running up and down the corridors, getting out of the train when the steam engine had to take on water, I just sat in my compartment, hidden away from everything and everybody.'

My mother had prepared Silvia so well for school that after her first year she skipped a class, which brought her to be just one year behind Enrico. Although I envied Enrico and Silvia going to school, I enjoyed my independence when they were away. I was envious of their closeness, and liked having my parents to myself. I was no longer The Titch. I felt so much bigger without them, and probably took advantage of my newly found confidence to boss around my dear friend and neighbour, Jenny.

For my lessons, my mother used books she received from a woman 'up-country' who organised correspondence courses. I remember devouring the *Old Lob* series. I became an avid reader.

I discovered Enid Blyton, starting with *Noddy* and moving on to the *Secret Seven* and the *Famous Five*. I learnt new words that represented a whole unfamiliar world of the English countryside: *robin* and *foxglove* and *stile* and *copse*. For years I mispronounced *dandelion* because I'd only ever seen the word in books, and never heard it spoken.

I enjoyed watching my mother clack-clack-clacking at her pedal sewing machine, making rompers for me from the leftovers of bright cotton dresses she made for herself. I loved standing on a stool helping her make pasta, squeezing the cool yellowish dough into long sheets through the rollers, and the sheets into strips through the cutters. I licked the bowl after she'd prepared her speciality, *il segreto della dama*, a no-bake cake made from melted chocolate, butter, egg yolks, crumbled Marie biscuits, and crushed peanuts, moulded into a large sausage, wrapped in kitchen paper and hardened in the fridge. I felt special when my father cut up my slice of buttered bread into 'exactly one hundred pieces' for my soup, and when, with surgical precision, he carved up a banana for me into a canoe, complete with seats and men with oars.

But sometimes I felt lonely, and dreamed of having a baby brother, someone I could care for, and who would have a close bond with me, like my siblings had. And if I had a baby brother, I would no longer be The Titch.

Although I enjoyed my relative independence, I missed Enrico and Silvia, and loved the excitement of them coming home for the holidays.

In the Doctor's Footsteps

My father was a man of many talents. Professionally, he turned his hand to whatever was required, in difficult environments, going way beyond general practice and his specialisation in Tropical Medicine.

Although all his brothers were doctors, he never encouraged any of us to take up medicine. Enrico hated the sight of blood, and seeing people suffer upset him. Silvia was much braver, and over the years often helped my father with his informal operations, when he'd remove people's lumps and bumps, or fix injuries. Needles were not a problem for her, and at school she was chief ear piercer, poking holes through girls' lobes with a needle that had been 'disinfected' under a hot tap, and assiduously instructing her patients to twist the thread daily.

As for me, apart from my short-lived wish to become a gynaecologist before I knew what that entailed, I never imagined that I could do anything scientific.

When I was seven, my father took me to watch him performing a Caesarean section. Standing on a chair, I had a prime viewpoint. I felt a little queasy as the scalpel cut into the dark flesh, and my father gently swabbed the blood that trickled out in a neat line;

I trembled with joy as a slimy baby boy was hoisted out, rubbed clean, and took his first breaths. I watched intently as the umbilical cord was cut, but found the long process of sewing up the mother's abdomen tedious, so I left before that was finished. The experience seemed miraculous to me: you start with one human being with a swollen belly, and half an hour later, you have two human beings. For many years, I was convinced that all babies were born in this way.

As District Medical Officer, my father would visit rural dispensaries, leaving an Indian assistant in charge of the Kigoma Hospital. We loved accompanying him on the trips north, because many places were accessible only by boat. The boat was called the *Kibisi*, and we could swim off it when it was moored.

Silvia recalls: 'Whenever the *Kibisi* anchored, we'd dive into the water. We discovered some enormous bivalves, which we pulled up from the sand deep down. Once we brought them home, and mamma cooked them, but they turned out to be inedible.'

The boat must have sailed close to Gombe Reserve, fifteen kilometres north along the lake, near the Burundi border, where primatologist Jane Goodall arrived in 1960 to carry out research on chimps. The Kenyan palaeontologist, Louis Leakey, had sent her. At the time she was in her twenties. Her ground-breaking work challenged the long-held ideas, that only humans could use tools, and that chimps were vegetarians. She observed distinctive characteristics in chimps, such as aggression and affection, and gave them all individual names.

A regular car trip was to Ujiji, a town of about 10,000 people, just a few kilometres south of Kigoma. Some European nuns had a large maternity centre there, and my father was often called in to help for difficult births.

Ujiji had been an important market centre during the slave trade, when local tribes would cross the lake and return with captives, who would then be sold and start the long trek to the

Indian Ocean. The physician, missionary and explorer David Livingstone campaigned tirelessly for the abolition of slavery. In a letter to the *New York Herald*, he wrote: ... *if my disclosures regarding the terrible Ujijian slavery should lead to the suppression of the East Coast slave trade, I shall regard that as a greater matter by far than the discovery of all the Nile sources together.*

In Ujiji, the journalist and explorer Henry Morton Stanley, sponsored by the *New York Herald*, found David Livingstone under a mango tree in 1871. There had been reports that Livingstone was lost, or even dead, and Stanley was sent to look for him. ... *I noticed he was pale, that he looked wearied and wan,* Stanley wrote in his book *How I found Livingstone in Central Africa.* ... *I did not know how he would receive me; so I ... walked deliberately to him, took off my hat, and said: 'Dr. Livingstone, I presume?'* There is some controversy over whether these words were actually spoken, as they do not appear in Stanley or Livingstone's diaries written at the time. A simple museum marks the spot today.

As a child I knew nothing of all this. I was vaguely aware that David Livingstone was both a doctor and a hero like my father, and that he had got lost, and was found in Ujiji.

Christmas in Kigoma

In my mind I see a misty cameo: a small girl stands on the lakeshore, with a group of four or five other children. She is wearing a bathing suit – clearly a hand-me-down, sagging from the straps at the top, and drooping down her skinny thighs. She is gazing out over the lake. It's warm, but the sky is cloudy.

A tiny dot appears on the horizon, and as it draws closer, the girl's heart starts pumping…

It's a motorboat, and in it stands a wobbling rotund white-bearded man wearing a red cloak and hat.

Did this really happen? Did Santa arrive at the Kigoma Club by boat? Enrico and Silvia have no recollection of it… how reliable are our memories? Have I simply constructed this image from my imagination?

The Christmas holiday was an exciting time. It was the longest of the three annual school holidays, and the end of the school year. Enrico and Silvia's good school reports were always a cause for celebration. I loved hearing all about their school adventures. It was wonderful to be a proper family again and have the house full. And with all the boarding school kids back, fancy dress parties were held at the club.

We always managed to find a scraggy fir to decorate with old baubles and bits of cotton wool. Christmas dinner consisted of tough roast chicken. Our *shamba* boy would chop off the heads of a couple of hens with a *panga*, and the hapless creatures would run around headless under the kapok trees in a final tragic dance.

Recently I was reminiscing with José Lamb, my parents' great friend from those days.

'Oh, chicken? What a luxury!' she said. 'I remember Colin and I went off on safari into the bush at Christmas. We were newlyweds and weren't tied down by children and school holidays. We hoped to shoot a guineafowl, and roast it like a turkey, but we had no luck. I think we had cheese on toast for our Christmas dinner.'

My parents tried to keep some Christmas traditions alive. We were allowed to stay up late on Christmas Eve to go to Midnight Mass at the local church. And there were gifts.

My first Christmas in Kigoma, when I was almost five, I was given a teddy bear to replace my old one, Panzotti, who had wire sticking out of his stomach and was deemed dangerous.

Although my new soft toy was bigger, softer, cleaner, and better in every way, I was deeply upset to have to say goodbye to my old Panzotti. My parents and siblings eventually managed to convince me to accept him.

'It's just his body that's changing. His soul is immortal,' they said. 'Inside he's the same Panzotti.' I came to love him dearly.

Panzotti's companion was a scruffy stuffed duck called Piopio. Although none of the three of us followed my father's footsteps into a medical career, playing doctors and nurses was one of our favourite games, and we always had the right gear.

That Christmas, Enrico and Silvia decided that although Panzotti clearly had a soul, Piopio didn't have a heart and needed one. They dressed up appropriately and set to work. With stethoscopes dangling around their necks, and wielding make-believe scalpels, they cut out a red heart shape from a piece of plastic, attached it to a small bell, and with great solemnity, performed the transplant, opening Piopio up with a pair of scissors, inserting the tinkling heart, and sewing him up again. I, being The Titch, was given an observer's role.

Sadly, Piopio was lost on a trip to Ujiji, but more than sixty years on, the 'new' Panzotti, now one-eyed, bruised, and battered, but together with his immortal soul, is still safely in the family.

The second Christmas in Kigoma brought a wonderful gift: my father made me a playhouse, complete with chimney, front door with a sliding bolt, and little shelves inside which folded up, hooking onto the walls to make more space. The notice on the front said Paola & Co. This was MY house, and everyone else was simply '& Co.'. Thirty years later, in Brussels, he built a similar house for our children.

On our third and last Christmas in Kigoma, a box arrived by train. It was stuffed with crisp, white polystyrene chips, like the snow we'd seen in London. In among the chips was the most wonderful gift: a 33 r.p.m. record of Bing Crosby's *A Christmas Sing with Bing*, with a picture on the sleeve of a smiling Bing sporting a bow tie, posing in front of a snowy globe. It was a compilation of songs by choirs from all over the world, with Bing introducing each one as though it were live. For years we loved imitating one track from it, a letter read by a young girl from Oklahoma: *Mah name is Dolores Short and Ah've lived in a children's home since Ah was a bye-bee*. The record has remained one of our unmissable family traditions ever since.

From our tropical verandah, where temperatures never dipped below the mid-twenties Centigrade, where every day and every night was guaranteed to be twelve hours long, where crickets and tree-frogs competed in cacophonous dusk concerts, and where our skies would open to the thunderous applause of tropical downpours, Bing transported us to 'real' Christmases from Salt Lake City to the Vatican, via the Netherlands, France, England and more, where children whose cheeks were pink from the cold, not from sunburn, wore coats and boots and gloves and hats, where Santa didn't arrive by motorboat but flew across the sky with reindeer and climbed down chimneys… and we dreamt of a world out there that seemed so much more exciting than our own.

Lake Tanganyika

Outside his work, my father had many interests, from astronomy, philosophy, and music to photography and carpentry.

As soon as we arrived in Kigoma, he started work on his masterpiece, a white catamaran with its two hulls held together by planks on which neat benches were mounted. The plywood for it had arrived in big crates on the train, goodness knows from where. He spent weeks working on it in our back garden. We called it *Spe*, an acronym of our three initials. My father told us that *spe* meant *hope* in Latin, and his hope was that it wouldn't sink. It seemed to me that he was displaying blind faith, rather than hope: how could he be sure that something so heavy would just sit on top of the water? He assured me that it was all to do with the air in the hulls, and water displacement, and that if he'd got his maths right, everything would be fine. When it was ready, we dragged it down to the lakeshore and launched it. It floated, and offered us many hours of joy. Enrico and Silvia were allowed to row, and I, being The Titch, sat in the middle.

We loved the lake. After all the years spent on Lake Victoria, it was a luxury to be able to swim with no fear of bilharzia. The Kigoma Club was a lakeshore shack, rather similar to the Musoma

Club we'd known, with a piece of water fenced off to make a swimming pool. The fence was full of holes, but it was supposed to keep fishing boats and crocodiles out.

This is where I learnt to swim, with the help of a red and white inflatable ball, which I clung on to for dear life. Enrico, who was an excellent swimmer, deflated the ball bit by bit, and my 'froggy legs', as my siblings called them, grew stronger and more efficient. After some weeks there was no air at all left in the ball, but I still insisted on clutching it to swim. Perhaps this is why later, when I started school, I found it so hard to learn to kick my legs properly for the crawl – I had thoroughly mastered my unique version of breast-stroke legs.

Enrico remembers one particular occasion in the lake: 'I was with mamma, swimming and chatting, when a water cobra popped his head and neck out of the water, looked at me and at mamma, and then ducked underwater again and swam off.' We saw snakes frequently in our various postings, and Enrico was an expert. 'Normally snakes don't bite if they are not provoked,' he told us. 'One rule: avoid being bitten by any snake: it may be poisonous.'

The Kigoma Club was the town's social hub. This is where the twenty-seven European families met up to have fun. It had a tennis court, and a bar area with tables and chairs where people held parties. Once, when Enrico and Silvia were away at school, my parents went to watch a film that was being projected there. This was presented to me as an exciting adventure: 'You'll get to sleep in the car!' The back seat of the VW was converted into a bed, complete with pillow and my teddy Panzotti, and I was tucked up and fast asleep by the time we got to the club. The car must have been parked all of ten metres from the outdoor screen, and I was no doubt lulled by the lapping of the waves on the lakeshore. A diligent night watchman came by and flashed an enormous torch onto my face from the side window, and I woke up, and screamed in terror. My parents rushed to see what had happened, and the experience was never repeated.

We were wild in those days, and it never occurred to anyone that the world outside our home might be dangerous. We explored freely. Silvia recalls that during the school holidays, 'I went with Enrico into the bush beyond our garden and set traps to catch birds. We'd get a cardboard box and prop it up and sprinkle crumbs near it. In theory, the birds were supposed to go for the bait, and we would wait for ages holding onto a string which would release the box... but we never caught a thing.'

Enrico learnt to make catapults at school with his friends, cutting Y-shaped sticks from small branches and rubber bands from inner tubes of car tyres, and fixing them together with leather strips. Fortunately, I don't think that method of bird-hunting was too successful either, but I was impressed by his craftsmanship, the power of his weapon, and the speed of the stones as he slung them far across the water into the lake.

The two of them were passionate about their stamp collection. Silvia remembers: 'Enrico and I would go knocking on strangers' doors and get great stamps. We'd also go scavenging in all the Indian *dukas*. Once we were looking for discarded envelopes in an enormous heap of papers behind a *duka*. We met someone who had been to Iraq and he gave us wonderful garish stamps.'

In the evenings, we often sat on the verandah and played cards or Scrabble. My mother taught us Italian card games – Scopa and Briscola – but our favourite was always Canasta, played with three packs. It took me years to discover that Enrico and Silvia used to fix the cards in advance to give me the best possible hand: they would giggle and nudge each other as I invariably won. The term 'Canasta closing face', meaning 'smug', has remained in the family.

From the verandah, we watched night fall in a flash, as it does near the equator, and the sunset lit up the Congo hills over the water. As night deepened, my father would point out the stars to us: 'Look, there are Sirius and Canopus. And those two are Alpha and Beta Centauri. They are the closest star system to us. And there's Orion's

Belt… see the three studs on it?' My favourite was the Southern Cross, which always hung its four corners like a hammock from its huge white Milky Way carpet. It made me feel safe.

Life was perfect. I had everything I needed… apart from a little brother, but with a bit of luck maybe, one day… I had family, friends, a natural playground stretching as far as the eye could see, and an entire lake. But as a six-year-old, little did I understand the trouble that was brewing on the other side of the water.

Like Lions

'*Come leoni,*' my mother said, her eyes wide, her hair dishevelled, and her crumpled cotton dress sweaty under the arms. 'They were like lions.'

It was an evening in November 1960. My mother was recounting her day to my father. I wondered what she meant by 'like lions'. That wasn't what I had seen. I had seen small boats landing on the shore by the Belbase, and white people struggling to get off with cases and bags and bundles. They were weak and whimpering and scruffy and scared. I had heard someone saying *fatigué*, which I knew meant tired.

The Belbase was a trading post on the lake, allowing for the transit of goods across Tanganyika and into Congo. Several Belgian families employed by the Belbase lived in Kigoma. Thanks to them, we picked up a smattering of French.

'As hungry as lions,' my mother continued. Ah yes. Now I understood. Hungry lions, not scary, fierce ones. I had spent the morning playing with my friends at the Belbase where my mother and the other European wives had been busy making sandwiches with fish paste from little glass jars and mashed boiled eggs mixed with mayonnaise, and piling them up on trays. And the Belgians from the boats – refugees, my mother called them – had gobbled them all up. Refugees, she said, are people who escape from wars, and there was a war across the lake in Congo.

'Will the war come here?' I asked.

'Don't worry,' my mother said, 'Tanganyika isn't like Congo. The local people here are peace-loving. And they like us. Papà helps them.'

The situation in Congo, just across the water from us, couldn't have been more different.

In the 1870s, about ninety years before my family lived in Kigoma, the Belgian King, Leopold II, had laid claim to the Congo. He hired Henry Morton Stanley to help him establish his authority there by negotiating with local leaders and building roads and a railway to facilitate trade. Stanley, after he had found Livingstone in 1872, had navigated the River Congo from the deep interior to the Atlantic.

At the Berlin Conference of 1884–1885, the colonial nations of Europe agreed to create what was called the Congo Free State, with Leopold as its head, on condition that this project improve the lives of the native inhabitants.

But what Leopold was interested in was making his fortune from ivory and rubber. The atrocities – and even genocide – committed during Leopold's reign are well documented and created an international scandal. Leopold was forced to hand the control of this personal treasure chest over to Belgian administration in 1908, and the Congo Free State was annexed as a Belgian colony called the Belgian Congo. Conditions improved slightly, but the priority still lay with promoting Belgian business and trade rather than developing the health and education sectors.

Belgian rule continued until 1960, when the country achieved independence after an impassioned nationalist movement. There had been little preparation for this massive upheaval, and the ensuing unrest and political violence continued for years.

Back in Kigoma, around the time of Congolese independence, our friend Colin Lamb, Inspector of Police for the Special Branch, was asked by the British administration to go over to Congo to assess the situation.

'I went with him,' his wife José told me. 'I used to love going over – Belgian-style cafés, baguettes, proper hairdressing salons – it was another world. I even had my hair done by a Belgian hairdresser. But you know, the Belgians weren't liked in Congo. They'd wear skimpy European clothes, and the local people disapproved. Colin's mission was to check up on the Force Publique and report back.'

The Force Publique was the police and military force, which had been set up by Leopold in 1885. At that time the officers were from various parts of Europe, and the soldiers under them were Africans from all over the continent, many of them mercenaries, others conscripted. During the Belgian colonial period, it became mostly Belgian officers and Congolese soldiers. They were formidable and brutal.

Five days after independence, just after José and Colin got back to Kigoma with the message that everything across the lake was fine, the soldiers mutinied against their white officers. The 100,000 Europeans still living in the country were terrified as violence spread, and started fleeing by whatever means they could.

That Christmas holiday, Enrico and Silvia came home from school two weeks early. 'They had to free up the schools,' Silvia recalls, 'so that the refugees could have somewhere to stay while repatriation was organised. I don't remember much about it, except that the next term we found a pair of red high-heeled shoes on top of a cupboard in our changing-room. We took turns tottering around in them.'

I was lucky to get first-hand accounts about the Belgian refugees from pupils of several Nairobi schools via our school Facebook page. Here are some of them:

I remember driving past the New Stanley Hotel in Nairobi with my parents and seeing refugees desperately trying to sell their cars and possessions. It was a sad sight.

*

It was late 1960. My father was a housemaster at the Prince of Wales School and some refugees were accommodated in the dorms there. I remember the children who had their pets with them – a kitten and an African Grey Parrot. The refugees looked so tired and confused, sitting in a group on the grass waiting to be told where to go. I was eight at the time.

*

I remember a refugee trying to get a room at the Norfolk Hotel for his family. He had a suitcase full of Belgian Congo money, which they would not accept. He stood in the reception with tears running down his face throwing money out of the suitcase and into the air.

*

The atrocities committed on Belgian 'colonials' and forced expropriation of their property began about six months earlier and caused them to flee – the women and children first. When we at Loreto were sent away before the end of term, my mother was helping with the refugees and I, just under fifteen, was asked to lend a hand as I was fairly good at French. I remember being in a huge hall where there were stacks of donated used clothes. Amidst the piles huddled pathetic little families – women and children only. One woman was hysterical and I was asked to try to find out what she wanted. It turned out to be serviettes hygiéniques *– sanitary towels. I shall never forget her distress and am to this* *day happy to have been able to help her, as of course these items, indispensable for a woman's dignity, were immediately procured for her, and for all the women.*

*

I remember hundreds of Belgian refugees in Kampala, their belongings in bundles. They looked broken and bewildered. Having later read the biography of Henry Morton Stanley and his role in helping the acquisitive King of the Belgians brutalise and enslave the peoples of the Congo, I could see the root of the anger of the Congolese, which had been festering for almost 100 years.

'You know, Paola,' José told me, 'my hairdresser was on one of those boats, terrified and bedraggled. I was shocked when I saw her clambering ashore. I couldn't believe it was the same woman I'd chatted with in her salon a few days before. She was lucky to escape. Many didn't.'

Kingdoms of Sand

My most vivid childhood memories come from our Kigoma days. Whenever I sit on a sandy shoreline, with waves lapping and ebbing around my thighs, I am drawn back to Lake Tanganyika, and to the castles I spent hours building.

I developed a special technique: the sand had to be of a specific wetness so that I could lift up a handful in my fingers, and allow it to drip, drip, drip in bulbous mini-mounds, and when a tower reached its maximum height before collapsing, I would make another beside it, and so on, till to me the whole construction looked like a magic kingdom as the grains of sand sparkled, drying and hardening in the sun, while I collected pebbles to decorate it. Across the water the hills of Congo shimmered in the blistering haze.

To me, Heaven couldn't be much better than this.

This was the period during which I began to feel independent, self-aware, responsible for my actions.

I learnt that I had a *soul*. In my mind, a soul was a shiny, white, oval mirror inside me, stretching the whole length of my abdomen, and I had to keep it clean if I was to get to Heaven. My soul was flexible, bending in the middle if I sat down. Any naughtiness would make a stain, which would have to be scrubbed off.

Did I create this image, or was it taught to me? My parents weren't particularly religious; once we were adults, my father often recounted that my mother 'saw the light' during her adolescence, 'like normal human beings', whereas it took him until he was thirty – husband, father of three, stuck on a remote island on the equator in the middle of Africa – to begin to have doubts about the strong beliefs of his childhood.

But despite this, my parents observed the rites of our religion. Were they giving it the benefit of the doubt? Was it a sort of Pascal's wager? The seventeenth-century theologian and philosopher Blaise Pascal argued that people should try to believe in God. If God doesn't exist, the losses are finite, whereas if He does, the gains are infinite, in the form of eternity in Heaven.

Perhaps my parents went through the motions, taking us to Mass on Sundays, respecting the 'no meat on Friday' rule (what a treat – we all loved fish!), through the steps of the Sacraments: Baptism, Holy Communion and Confirmation, because that was the way things had been done for generations in their families… or maybe they simply wanted to ensure we didn't stand out from others in our schools and social circles.

I received my First Holy Communion in Kigoma. I don't remember much about the preparation, apart from going to catechism classes. Perhaps it was there that I learnt about souls. I was six, and my parents wanted me to have both Communion and Confirmation under my belt before I went to boarding school the following year. A spotless soul was required for anyone receiving First Holy Communion, so I, along with all the other First Communicants, would have to go to Confession, which meant kneeling in a darkened confessional – a sort of sentry-box with a partition to separate the penitent from the priest. I would have to say, 'Bless me, Father, for I have sinned. This is my first confession.' And then I would tell him my sins and he would give me Penance in the form of prayers to say. That last part seemed easy: I liked saying prayers, although it did seem odd to me that the one to the Virgin Mary started with the words 'Hail Mary, full of grapes'.

I remember my parents talking Confession through with me. I couldn't think of anything I'd done that would qualify as a sin, apart from once refusing to eat my soup.

'Just tell the priest you've been a good girl,' my mother said, but that felt like a bit of a copout, and didn't match the format I'd learnt, so in that dark, scary confessional, I told him a) that I had been disobedient – I reckoned having rejected the soup might justify this, and b) that I had told a lie – in case the soup incident wasn't bad enough, or perhaps disobedience wasn't a sin that left a stain on your soul, in which case I had lied to him. Another complication was that my father, in an uncharacteristic gesture, had smacked my bottom for not eating the soup. This was the only time he ever smacked me; a bitter humiliation, because we had been invited to lunch at the home of friends, and the punishment was meted out in front of them. So I had already suffered doubly for my sin.

The priest told me to say three Hail Marys and one Our Father as Penance, after which my soul was sparkling and I was able to dress up in a beautiful long white dress made from embossed satin fabric that my maternal grandmother had sent for the occasion. Did I really believe that the Host was the Body of Christ? I think I did, and I was careful to swallow it whole, so as not to hurt Him with my teeth.

Recently I asked Enrico and Silvia what their feelings were about religion when they were small.

'I believed that having Communion meant taking Jesus into my body,' Enrico said. 'I remember Confession at school and having difficulty in finding naughty things. A classic when we got older was "having impure thoughts". That was considered bad: not a "venial" but a "mortal" sin… We had Mass every day at school, except when we skipped it by hiding in the cupboards.' (Wasn't that worthy of confessing, I wonder?)

Silvia said, 'Confession was always a problem because I was such a goody goody. Before Confession I would try to tell a lie. But once I found a tennis ball behind the courts and I stole it. I could have found the owner but I wanted to keep the tennis ball. Now I had a problem because this was a real sin. It took me a year to confess it, by which time I had lost the ball. After all the angst the priest said, "Say three Hail Marys." I was so shocked that it was such a small penance for a big sin that I thought maybe he hadn't heard me, but I didn't have the courage to tell him again.'

Although we never discussed these things at the time, we all went through similar thought patterns, even through to our late teenage rejection of almost everything that had been inculcated in us.

But some elements remain, and I believe that this world holds heaven-sent experiences: like cooking with a granddaughter propped up on a stool beside me, discussing the merits of purple versus blue mixing bowls; or the first time her baby sister looks at me, captures my gaze, and breaks into a smile which says, 'I know you; you're my Nonna'.

Last summer, I was on an unusually sunny beach in North Antrim with my four grandsons. They were sitting on the shoreline, the waves lapping at their feet, lifting handfuls of sand, which were drip, drip, dripping into small hillocks, one beside the other. Instinctively, I started collecting little shiny pebbles, which they carefully placed on the walls of their castles. 'Look, Nonna, we have a whole kingdom!' one said. Across the water the hills of the Mull of Kintyre glistened… and I said a silent prayer that the world still held a few of these moments for me.

Heaven couldn't be much better.

NAIROBI AND MWANZA

1961-1963

A Speck of Dust

We watched the taxi cruise down the bougainvillea-lined avenue, turn right at the main road, turn right again at the top of the hill, and disappear towards Nairobi airport. It was October 1961, my first day at Loreto Convent Msongari. I was seven and three-quarters.

After my father's posting to Kigoma had ended, we'd spent several months on long leave in Italy, which is why we were joining school halfway through the final term of the year. My parents were now heading to Mwanza, Tanganyika's second-largest town, on the southern shore of Lake Victoria, which would be our home for the next two years. My father had received a promotion and was to be Provincial Medical Officer.

We had dropped Enrico off at St. Mary's School, next door. He'd run off to join his friends, and the taxi had driven us down the short tree-lined driveway between the schools. It was so different from our scruffy Kigoma garden: everything was fresh and green and manicured.

Mother Superior had welcomed us in the Parlour, a small sitting room at the front of the main school building. The Parlour, I soon learnt, was a special place, and that was the only time that

I set foot in it. We drank milky tea and munched Marie biscuits, and my parents talked to Mother Superior for a long time, their words drifting above my head. When they'd finished, they quickly hugged and kissed us, and were gone. Were those tears I saw in my mother's eyes?

And now here I was, clutching Silvia's hand. I felt like a speck of dust in an enormous new world. We were wearing our uniforms: navy blue tunic, white blouse, red tie, long red sash with tassels at the end called a *girdle*, red blazer with the school crest, navy boater hat, white ankle socks and shiny black shoes. Silvia had spent a long time teaching me how to fashion the knot in my tie and girdle.

She squeezed my hand. 'C'mon, Titch,' she said. 'I'll show you around.'

We passed the Hall, a big building with a jacaranda tree dominating it at the front. Mauve blossom carpeted the ground, and a honey scent filled the cool dry air. 'That's where we have plays and concerts, and films on Sundays, and Assembly when it's raining,' Silvia said, pushing open the door. I'd never seen such an enormous stage.

The big space in front of the Parlour, Silvia told me, was called the Front of the House, and we weren't allowed to walk across it except on Sundays between four and six o'clock, which was Visiting Time, when boys from St. Mary's would come to see their sisters. Oh, it would be lovely to see Enrico once a week, I thought. I was already guessing that I wouldn't see Silvia much during the week, so at least on Sundays we'd be almost a proper family. 'The Big Girls can see other boys, but only with written permission from their parents,' Silvia said. 'And if you get in trouble, you have to go to Detention at Visiting Time.'

She led me to the Chapel, and we peeped inside.

It smelt of incense, and was bright and airy. A couple of nuns, heads bent and hands joined in prayer, knelt on kneelers placed around the sides of the long bench pews. I spotted the Confessional, and a shiver ran through me. We passed the dining room, which smelt musty and metallic. Silvia pointed to another big building: 'St. Joseph's. That's where the Big Girls sleep. They get rooms for two or three people, not dorms.'

Behind St. Joseph's were the playing fields: murram hockey, netball and rounders pitches, and an area covered with trees. Here and there, groups of girls played hopscotch, or sat on the grass chatting. We stopped to stare at a thick column of safari ants crossing the path. We were used to seeing them in Kigoma, but never so many together. We stepped over them gingerly: those ants had a fierce bite.

A heavy metal gate led to a square of buildings around manicured lawns. 'The Quadrangle,' Silvia said. Quadrangle. A big name for a big place. 'See where the paths cross in the middle? If you get caught talking after lights out, you might get sent to stand there for hours, and I tell you, it's cold at night!'

I gazed around at the arched verandahs. This is where I would spend the next ten or so years of my life, with three brief breaks at home for holidays each year. A loud, dull sound coming from further down the corridor interrupted my reverie. *Clang* – pause – *clang–clang–clang*. 'The nuns' gong,' Silvia said. 'That's how the nuns are called. Every nun has a number. One and then three is thirteen. Gerty – Mother Gertrude – I think.'

She led me up a flight of stairs to the upper floor. 'These are the junior dorms. Let's find your name.' She scanned the list on each door till she found it. 'Here you are.' We found the one unmade bed, with clean sheets folded on it. 'Mattress is a bit lumpy. If you get here before the others at the beginning of term you can bag a good mattress. I'll have a rotten one this term too.'

We continued past the dorms till we reached an alcove with a statue of Jesus at the end, and a shiny floor. 'This used to be our Chapel,' Silvia said, 'but now that we have a new one, the Prods use this one.'

We turned along another verandah. A nun passed us, her heavy rosary beads jangling around her waist. 'Good afternoon, Mother Miriam,' Silvia said, placing one foot behind the other and bobbing down. The nun passed by. 'That was Minnie. A bit fierce, but kind. You'll have to learn to curtsey, Titch. Forgot to teach you.' She showed me the bathrooms, eight of them, with lists on the doors. 'You sign up here for your weekly bath. Here are the toilets. These are the science labs. They're kept locked.' We passed a glass-fronted cabinet, in which were displayed holy pictures, rosaries and statues. 'And this is the Holy Press. Mother Teresa – Tickie – looks after it, and you can buy holy pictures and statues here.' We moved on. 'This is the infirmary where you go if you're sick.'

And on we went along the third side, past more dorms. 'Out of bounds,' Silvia whispered, indicating the fourth side. 'That's where the nuns sleep.'

I followed Silvia downstairs, and our tour continued, around the ground floor. 'This is the changing room for Standards One to Four,' she said. 'You'll be in here.' I was to be in Standard Two. We passed classrooms, the Nurse's Room, and the Office. 'You get sent to the Office if you do something bad...' We went out through another set of gates to the tennis courts, Art Room, and clear azure swimming pool. A group of girls of around my age were swimming laps. Thank goodness Enrico had taught me how to swim... but that high diving board at the end looked scary...

Silvia led me back into the Quad, where a group of three or four girls were sitting on a low wall swinging their legs. 'I'll have to go now,' she said. 'I'll come and check on you when I can.' She turned to a tall, athletic girl with thick chestnut hair, olive skin, eyes that were deep and dark and twinkly, and a big smile. 'You're Val, right? Standard Two? Doreen's cousin? This is my kid sis, Paola. She's new. Could you look after her?'

I held back my tears. My head spun. I couldn't decide whether I was excited or terrified. This was like what I'd read in the Malory

Towers books, only it was real. I had to learn to find my way about. I couldn't depend on Silvia. But I knew she would always be there if I needed her.

'Titch, you'll be fine.'

She gave me a hug and was gone.

Blending In

Val took me under her wing. She was taller than I by about a head, and confident: I was happy to shelter in her shadow.

That first day, by the wall in the Quad, she taught me how to curtsey. I followed her to my first class.

'I'm Mrs. Mac,' the teacher said. She had a soft face, and looked like a granny. 'Mrs. McKeown, really, but that's too hard to say.'

I sat down beside Val. The first lesson was art.

'Today we're drawing ducks on a river,' Mrs. Mac said. When I had managed a river by drawing two parallel blue lines across my page with a ruler, tears started welling in my eyes, and soon they were dripping onto the paper.

'What's the matter, pet?'

'I don't know how to draw a duck,' I sobbed. My mother had taught me to read and write and count and add and take away, and I knew how to colour in pictures neatly, but we had never done much drawing.

Mrs. Mac took my pencil and drew a wide figure two. From the top left end of the two, she fashioned a pointy beak, then swooped around clockwise in a half-circle to join the bottom right side. A small circle for an eye, a wide U for a wing, and miraculously, there was my duck.

'See, pet, it's not so hard.'

My drawing skills never developed much further, but I will always be grateful to Mrs. Mac.

I soon got used to the school routine: wakeup bell, prayers, Mass, breakfast, class, break, class, lunch, class, prep, playtime, prayers, supper, prayers, bed.

We had swimming first period once a week. Nairobi is situated at almost 1,800 metres above sea level – that's a good 400 metres higher than the top of Ben Nevis. Although the middle of the day was hot, early mornings were cold, much colder than Kigoma had been... perhaps twelve or thirteen degrees. At my first swimming lesson, I jumped in – the others could all dive head first – and swam a length as fast as I could. 'Frog legs!' someone teased, and I felt the wet warmth of a blush rising from my middle to my face. I soon mastered proper breaststroke legs, and Val helped me learn to dive.

We small boarders were under the care of a slim, grey-haired woman called Mrs. Scott. She was strict, but not unkind. On our first evening, I followed Val and the rest of the girls into our dressing room, where we were to change into our pyjamas, which we each kept in a little cabinet. Tired after all the excitement of the day, I stripped off down to my pants.

'Paola Fornari!' Mrs. Scott scolded. She pronounced it *Fanari*. 'And you, a doctor's daughter! What are you doing? You must learn to undress modestly!' I looked around. Forty girls stopped what they were doing and stared at me. One or two giggled. I saw that everyone else was skilfully manoeuvring the changing operation hunched forwards with their dressing gowns balanced on their shoulders. I couldn't understand what being a doctor's daughter had to do with it, but that was far from the only time the reprimand was used against me at Loreto.

Every evening we washed our faces and brushed our teeth in the mould-and-chlorine-smelling bathrooms, and lined up to be checked by Mrs. Scott, who would look at our necks and pull our ears to inspect behind them. At first I regularly failed the quality control test. 'Back you go!' Mrs. Scott would say. 'Your neck isn't clean.' And I would scrub and scrub with my face flannel. After a few days I realised Mrs. Scott was mistaking the two moles on the side of my neck, now doubled in size thanks to the harsh treatment they had received, for blobs of dirt. Those moles still flare up from time to time.

My mother had provided me with pink Lifebuoy soap, which she considered a good disinfectant. It stank. Lifebuoy was about the least cool soap on the planet, and I had to suffer smothered titters from the others. I soon learnt that the best means of survival was to blend in. From my second term onwards, I managed to persuade my mother to buy heaven-scented Imperial Leather or curiously transparent Pears.

Before bed we would brush our hair, with a hundred strokes of the brush and twenty of the comb counted out in unison.

In the morning we would repeat the washing, changing and brushing routine. The changing room always smelt of ammonia. 'You're not allowed to say anything about it,' Val told me. 'It's Lindy. She wets her bed. It's not her fault. It's like an illness.'

Playtime was wonderful. After prep we could change into our home clothes, put on aprons, and go out to the vast wooded area beside the sports fields. Apart from the classic hopscotch, I learnt French skipping: two girls would stand about a metre apart with an elastic wound around their legs, and another would go through a series of complicated jumps in the middle. As the game progressed, the elastic would be raised, to make it more difficult. Skipping with a rope was great fun too, and involved a lot of chants:

Father Christmas lost his whiskers
How many whiskers did he lose?

And the rope would be twirled faster and faster as we all chanted *one, two, three...*

British Bulldogs was a rougher game, which involved running across a field and trying not to get caught by the 'bulldogs' in the middle. It often ended with torn dresses.

If ever we were unwell, we had to go and see the nurse, who was an elderly dragon. She had three remedies: Algipan (which smelt like Lifebuoy soap), used to treat anything from an insect bite to a twisted ankle, gargle for sore throats, and a thick foul-tasting mud-coloured concoction for everything else. 'Down the hatch!' she'd chirp as she handed out the mixture in a small plastic goblet.

Learning manners was part of the fitting in process. At breakfast we were taught to cut our toast neatly into four triangles, and to chop the top off our boiled eggs, rather than cracking them on the table and peeling them as we did at home.

Mealtimes were great. I enjoyed the food, apart from a variety of milk puddings: semolina, tapioca, and coconut custard, which we used to call 'Matthias's Toenails'. We had a love-hate relationship with Matthias, who was the boss of the kitchen staff, at once friendly but fierce, with black teeth filed into points.

At mealtimes the post was distributed... blue air letters arrived every week for us with news from Mwanza.

On Saturdays we had Letter Writing. We would all sit in a classroom with our pencils and writing pads, and as the nun on duty wrote on the board, we copied:

Dear Mummy and Daddy,
How are you? I am very well. Thank you for your letter.
Last week we watched a film. It was called...

At the end of the letter, we were allowed to express our own ideas – up to a point – everything was checked when we'd finished.

I hated writing 'Mummy and Daddy'. My parents were *mamma* and *papà*, and I felt I was writing to strangers. But I didn't dare complain.

Was I homesick? I don't think so. I focussed on learning new skills, such as cleaning my shoes and making my bed with hospital corners and keeping my socks rolled up in pairs (as well as drawing ducks, changing discreetly, and chopping the tops off boiled eggs), and spent a lot of energy trying not to attract attention.

But I tripped up a few times. Once was in my first week. After class, we were allowed to take four sweets, which Mrs. Scott would hand out from our personal tuck boxes. It was the highlight of our day. One afternoon, I saw a girl called Molly take her box to the back of the crowd of girls out of Mrs. Scott's sight, and empty dozens of sweets into the oversized pocket of her apron. My hand shot up.

'Mrs. Scott! Molly took lots of sweets!'

The room hushed, and yet again, everyone stared. Molly was called to the front of the group and sent to the headmistress.

Val put her arm around me and said, 'You have to learn not to tell tales. Ever.'

I often wonder whether Molly remembers that incident. I don't know who suffered more in its aftermath: Molly or I.

But I learnt.

Rituals and Illness

Dong... dong... dong... The chapel bell chimed. Val and I were walking across the Quad with a few other girls and a nun, Tickie. We stopped in our tracks. The hot sun was beating directly overhead. Two more groups of three peals, then a series of nine peals.

'*The Angel of the Lord declared unto Mary,*' recited Tickie.

'*And she conceived by the Holy Ghost,*' the girls responded in unison. I mumbled in embarrassment. And then everyone launched into '*Hail Mary...*' At least I knew that part and had learnt that it was '*full of grace*', not '*grapes*'.

This routine was called the Angelus. The bells chimed three times a day, at six in the morning, when we were still in bed, at noon, and at six in the evening. Apart from in the first Angelus of the day, we had to stand still and pray whenever we heard the bells.

We had a short Mass every morning before breakfast, Confession on Saturdays, and a long Mass with several hymns on Sundays. For Sunday Mass we dressed up in white frocks. All Masses were in Latin. On Fridays we went to Chapel for the Stations of the Cross. Fourteen simple pictures around the Chapel walls depicted Christ's struggle as he carried his cross up Calvary. We stopped at each one and said a prayer. I particularly liked the station in which Veronica wiped Christ's face… *what a loving thing to do*, I thought.

We had Grace before and after every meal (I thought '*Blessed be God*' was '*Bless me, God*'), prayers, rosary and a ceremony called Benediction every evening in the chapel. Before lights out, we kneeled by our beds and prayed. One prayer was scary:

Now I lay me down to sleep,
I pray the Lord my soul to keep,
And if I die before I wake,
I pray the Lord my soul to take.

Why might I die before I wake? I was not even eight. How would the Lord take my soul out of me? Where would he take it?

I preferred the one that went:

Goodnight, Jesus, I'm going to bed,
Work is over, prayers are said,
I'm not afraid of the dark or the night,
For You will watch till morning light.

(For years I thought the last line was '*till morning is night*'.)

In that first term I learnt a lot of prayers. Indulgences were a favourite of mine: little invocations you could say to shorten the time you'd need to spend in Purgatory when you died, if your soul wasn't clean enough for you to go straight to Heaven. We had a booklet that listed the prayers and the length of the reduced sentence: for example, if you said '*Jesus, Mary, and Joseph, I give you my heart and my soul*', you got a rebate of seven days. I remember repeating those words, counting on my fingers, multiplying by seven, and clocking up hundreds, even thousands, of days.

Despite the new prayer routine being so intensive and unfamiliar, it didn't faze me: I found it comforting. It marked the day into chunks, and gave the whole week a regular, predictable pattern.

Occasionally we'd leave the grounds in the rickety green school bus, to go to a music festival, or to attend a sports day or play at another school, with Michael the driver at the wheel in his smart peaked hat, and a nun in attendance. The bus couldn't make it up the steep hill at the end of the avenue, so we would all pile out and climb to the top. Once we were back in, we'd say a prayer to St. Christopher to keep us safe, and then go into endless Litanies, the nun leading, and the girls responding in unison:

Nun: *Virgin most merciful,*
Girls: *Pray for us.*
Nun: *Virgin most faithful,*
Girls: *Pray for us.*
Nun: *Mirror of justice,*
Girls: *Pray for us.*
Nun: *Seat of wisdom,*
Girls: *Pray for us.*
Nun: *Cause of our joy,*
Girls: *Pray for us...*

... and dozens more similar petitions.

It took me a while to catch on that the giggling Big Girls at the back of the bus were responding '*Pray for the bus*'... perhaps not such a bad idea.

I did not question the seemingly senseless words. It was simply a reassuring murmur washing over me, back and forth, like the ebb and flow of waves.

'God will give you anything you want,' the nuns told us. 'As long as what you want is a good thing, and you're a good girl. All you have to do is pray to Him.'

There was only one thing I wanted. For years I had dreamed of having a baby brother, someone I could look after while Enrico and Silvia played together, and who would grow up to be my playmate. But it had not happened. Dreaming was perhaps not as good as praying, I decided, so I spent a lot of my first term praying to God, Jesus, Mary, and all the Saints for my wish to come true. I tried to behave. Surely a baby brother was a good thing to pray for.

I looked forward to the Christmas holidays. Enrico, Silvia and I would spend two days and two nights on the train and steamer, travelling to our new home in Mwanza, almost 700 kilometres away. And if everything went according to plan, I'd find a baby brother waiting for me.

A week before the end of that first term, along with a few other girls, I became ill. An itchy rash, which spread from behind my ears to my neck and then all over my body, soon followed a runny nose, sore eyes and fever, and I was sent to the infirmary. It was measles. The infirmary, which had eleven beds, was soon full, and two or three nearby dormitories were requisitioned to accommodate more patients as the virus spread. In the infirmary we prayed a lot to St. Roch, the patron saint of sick people. I liked his name: it invoked strength and stability. He was Rocco in Italian: even better.

The infirmary was boring. Fortunately, I wasn't seriously ill, but the curtains were closed to keep out the light, and we weren't allowed to read. Through the windows, we could hear excitement mounting for the end of term, with girls chanting:

No more Latin, no more French,
No more sitting on a hard, old bench,
No more spiders in my tea,
Making googly eyes at me.

In the evenings, as the boarders gathered around the Crib in a corner of the Quad, the echo of their voices rose up to us:

> *Come, come, come to the manger,*
> *Children, come to the children's King;*
> *Sing, sing,*
> *Chorus of angels,*
> *Stars of morning, o'er Bethlehem sing.*
>
> *He lies 'mid the beasts of the stall,*
> *Who is Maker and Lord of us all,*
> *The wintry wind blows cold and dreary,*
> *See, He weeps, the world is weary,*
> *Lord, have pity and mercy on me.*

I loved the chorus, but the end of that first verse seemed miserable: quite apt for my plight.

What stirred me the most was the sound that floated up to us of girls singing the Holiday Hymn: it made sense. We'd worked hard and we deserved a holiday. That particular hymn still brings goose pimples to my skin.

> *Mother of all that is pure and glad, all that is bright and blest,*
> *As we have taken our toil to thee, so we will take our rest.*
> *Take thou and bless our holiday, O causa nostrae laetitiae!*

Petronella, a Big Girl in the bed opposite mine, had a transistor radio. I remember imagining an alien world as she sang along to 'English Country Garden':

> *How many kinds of sweet flowers grow*
> *In an English country garden*
> *I'll tell you now of some that I know*
> *And those that I miss you'll surely pardon*
> *Daffodils, hearts ease and phlox*
> *Meadowsweet and lady smocks*

Gentians, lupins and tall hollyhocks
Roses, foxgloves, snowdrops, forget-me-nots
In an English country garden

When we'd lived in England for six months, our English country garden had been slushy snow under a thick blanket of fog.

A much more inspiring song which beat out from Petronella's radio was Helen Shapiro's 'Walking Back to Happiness'. It was jolly and strong and looked optimistically to the future.

Silvia had to stay behind at school to wait for me to get better, and we travelled home together by plane two days after the end of term. I often wonder how the logistics of these travel permutations were worked out.

Michael, together with Minnie, drove us to the airport in the school car... definitely a few notches above the green bus. I had lost weight and felt weak, and was disappointed to have missed the train and boat adventure, but as Minnie prayed to St. Christopher, and I clutched Silvia's hand in the back seat, I could feel my heart beating with joy...

Helen Shapiro's deep voice rang in my head:
Walking back to happiness, woopah oh yeah yeah...
We were going home!

An Antelope
and Other Creatures

Tanganyika had become independent on 9th December 1961, just a few days before the Christmas holidays started. The transition had been peaceful, and we noticed little change, apart from the flag and the anthem, a Swahili version of the rousing South African hymn '*Nkosi Sikelel' iAfrika*', so now, instead of singing 'God Save our Gracious Queen' at official events or at the cinema, we sang '*Mungu Ibariki Afrika*' – God Bless Africa – the only national anthem in the world that still gives me goose bumps.

But in our new home in Mwanza, in December 1961, Tanganyika's independence was the last thing on my nearly-eight-year-old mind. There was a more important issue to resolve. My prayer for a baby brother had not been answered. I needed to know why.

I approached my father, hands on hips, and asked him. He sat down beside me, a blank piece of paper in front of him on the dining-room table, a sharpened pencil in his hand. In his customary meticulous way, he drew the outline of a woman's body, and in the middle, just above where the legs joined, he added what looked like an antelope's head, with horns curling down and inwards. Each horn had a round ball at the bottom.

'This is the inside of a woman's body,' he said, his voice, as always, soft. 'That big triangle in the middle is called the uterus. The round balls are ovaries. In there, eggs are made which then travel around these tubes to the uterus and sometimes they grow into babies.'

He didn't provide further details about when the 'sometimes' might be, nor did he say how the babies got out. At this stage I still thought it was via Caesarean, like in the operation I had watched him perform in Kigoma.

'Sometimes the ovaries get sick,' he continued, 'and a doctor has to take them out. It happened to mamma when you were very small, and that's why she can't have another baby. Her body doesn't make eggs any more.' He didn't mention that when all this happened, my mother had been pregnant and had lost the baby who would have been my little brother. He just smiled. 'But we are lucky, because you three were born before that, and we have a lovely big family which is just fine as it is.'

I clutched my churning stomach, and squeezed my eyes shut. How was it possible? The nuns had promised. Jesus had performed all sorts of miracles, like turning water into wine so as not to disappoint people at a party. Surely my request was far simpler and more useful? How could my father, who knew everything, be contradicting what the nuns had said? And why had God not kept my mother's ovaries healthy?

Anger followed disappointment. Up to this point, I had thought adults were infallible. They were powerful. They told the truth. And now I had been let down by all the adults who were supposed to look after me. And by God and Jesus and Mary and all the Saints.

I thought for a while and decided there was no more I could do. Clearly there had been an error in The Plan somewhere along the line. The baby brother idea, which had occupied my thoughts and prayers for years, was shelved, for ever.

I turned to other matters and ran off to find Enrico and Silvia: we had some exploring to do.

Our house in Mwanza was on a rocky outcrop called Capri Point, overlooking the Bismarck Rock on Lake Victoria. Two central rooms were surrounded by verandahs, which had been sealed with netting to keep the mosquitoes out. These makeshift spaces became our breezy bedrooms. On the walls, geckos scuttled, their lightning tongues flicking. Sometimes you could discern eggs inside their translucent abdomens. *Their ovaries are okay*, I remember thinking.

Our garden was, once again, scrubland and trees. Hyraxes gambolled over the rocks in their dozens: these short-tailed creatures, about the size of rabbits, have long tusk-like incisors and, along with sea-cows, are the elephant's closest relatives. In those days they were hunted for their soft skins. I made no connection between the cute furry animals and the soft, patchwork blankets sold by the roadside… it's so easy now to say 'those were different times'.

It was in Mwanza that my father built us the first of many treehouses. Troops of monkeys would leap between the tree and the corrugated iron roof of our house, and, unaware of the danger they posed – they could become aggressive if they felt threatened, though ours seemed quite tame – we would feed them bananas. In a letter to my maternal grandparents, my brother wrote: *You need to know that monkeys come and pay us visits every single day and each of us children has a favourite monkey. Mine is one with a mumps-like face, different from all the other monkeys I've seen (and I've seen many), and a son who hasn't yet learnt to walk so he's always attached to his mother.*

Our friends José and Colin Lamb followed us from Kigoma to Mwanza, with their first child, a daughter. Colin had left the police and was now in the Game Department, where one of his tasks was to relocate wild animals. 'You see, Paola,' José told me recently, 'the balance had to be right. If too many leopards were killing baboons, or if you had too many lions in one area, they had to be moved elsewhere. They'd capture them. I remember a lion roaring from his cage, banging his nose against the bars, while the baby was sleeping nearby in her pram… terrifying!'

In our garden, agama lizards would pose on rocks, scarlet heads and puffed chests raised up by their forearms, cobalt bodies trailing behind them. Monitor lizards, which could reach two metres in length, were less common, and well camouflaged as they basked in the sunshine. They would startle us by scurrying away if we disturbed them. José remembers them as 'little dragons'. We used to call them iguanas, and it was only decades later that I learnt that iguanas are not found in Africa.

I often wonder how my mother settled in to new places, moving hundreds of kilometres every couple of years, having to make new friends. My father simply slotted into his busy role in whatever hospital was assigned to him and loved what he was doing. I never remember my parents complaining, though it can't have been easy for them to integrate into the mostly British society they mixed with in Tanganyika. However, through my father's quiet professionalism and my mother's sociability, they managed to build a reputation and integrate.

Where was 'home' for our family? My parents had dived blindly into British-administered Tanganyika not long after the end of the Second World War, at a time when the British did not view Italians in a positive light. I never felt any sense of national pride emanating from my parents. My father, in particular, seemed almost ashamed of his country and its chaos. He had always admired the British, their organisation, and their style. He often spoke of his first encounter with British people at the end of the war.

'When the Allies arrived, we were overjoyed. We befriended two British soldiers, a sergeant from Lancashire and a sapper from Kent. We kept in touch for many years after the war. Such gentlemen.'

Our parents never had any particular language 'policy' for us. We spoke whatever language surrounded us: English 'socially' and at school, and Swahili with local people. At home we gradually morphed from Italian to a mixture of Italian and English with a smattering of Swahili. English soon became our dominant language, and that is the language in which Enrico, Silvia and I have always communicated.

We weren't considered 'expats': back then the term generally referred to diplomats or people who had been sent abroad to work for an international organisation. And though many of our school friends were 'settlers', we didn't fit into that category either. I suppose you could call us economic migrants, though my parents had never intended to stay in Tanganyika for ever. We children didn't feel 'properly' Italian: we were simply part of a community of Europeans who were working in East Africa.

And those are the people we identify with most, even now, whatever nationality is on their passport. They are the ones who understand when we talk about dogs mauled by leopards and swimming lions and favourite monkeys.

For now, Mwanza was home. It was a metropolis, after Kigoma. There was a large European community. There were even two Rolls Royces, belonging to wealthy Indian brothers called Chopra, one a doctor and one a businessman, and Enrico was delighted to once manage to hitch a lift in one.

From Capri Point, we three could stroll down a dusty track to the Club, much more sophisticated than the one in Kigoma, which had a jukebox with crackly speakers, and a kidney-shaped swimming pool where we spent many happy hours.

Enrico had a friend called Keith Carrott. He had bright red hair and freckles, and I thought he was the most handsome creature God had ever created. Like Enrico, he was twelve, and I don't think he ever spoke to me. But I was in love. What did 'being in love' mean for a nearly-eight-year-old? Terror every time I saw him, embarrassment in case Enrico or Silvia noticed, and a warm fuzzy feeling running through my whole body every time I thought of him.

Other, safer friends filled our lives. I remember once walking with Silvia to the home of a girl called Gabriella. She must have been thirteen, and she'd just come back from Italy where she'd learnt to do the Twist, which had become all the rage. She put Chubby Checker's 'Let's Twist Again' on her turntable and gave us a demonstration. 'Rub your back with a towel,' she said, as she stood with her feet shoulder-width apart, rotating her hips, arms punching back and forth. Silvia and I watched, gobsmacked. 'Stamp out a cigarette!' And her foot tapped as she lunged forwards, backwards, swivelled from side to side, and bobbed up and down. Silvia and I certainly earned kudos from this private demo when we got back to school.

That first Christmas in Mwanza was disappointing. We received many gifts, but I paid little heed to most of them. What bothered me were the records. Enrico was given a beautiful Elvis Presley LP. Silvia received a Cliff Richard EP album. Cliff was nothing to envy; people (or at least, the kids we knew) were divided into Elvis or Cliff fans, and we were firmly in the Elvis camp. My gift? A Mantovani SP record. I tried to hide my bitterness. I'd survived my first term (well, half term) at school; I'd survived measles… and what did I have to show for it? Two measly tracks by Mantovani. I'd never even heard of him.

Time to go back to school. At least I'd not have to face Keith Carrott, but would be able to daydream about him – by the end of the holiday he had replaced all the brain-space that had previously been occupied by my longing for a baby brother – and I could scribble KC on my exercise books without Enrico and Silvia knowing…

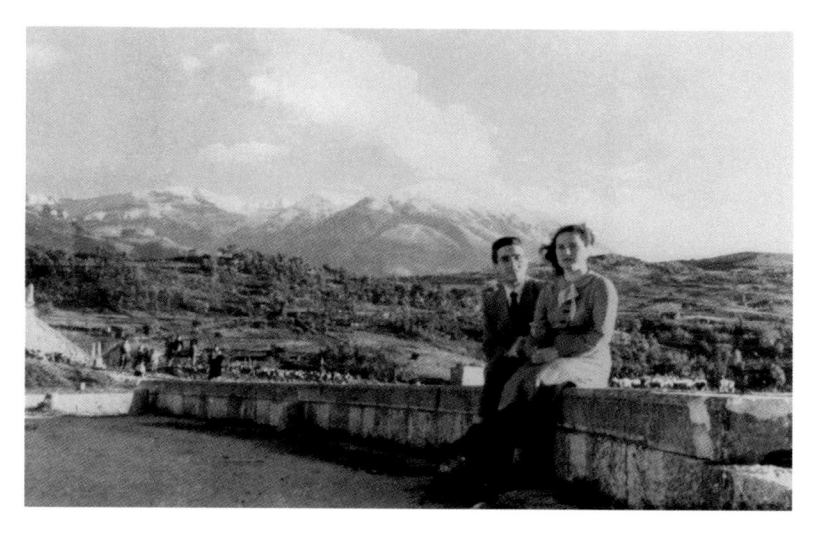

Papà and zia Teta, Abbateggio, 1947

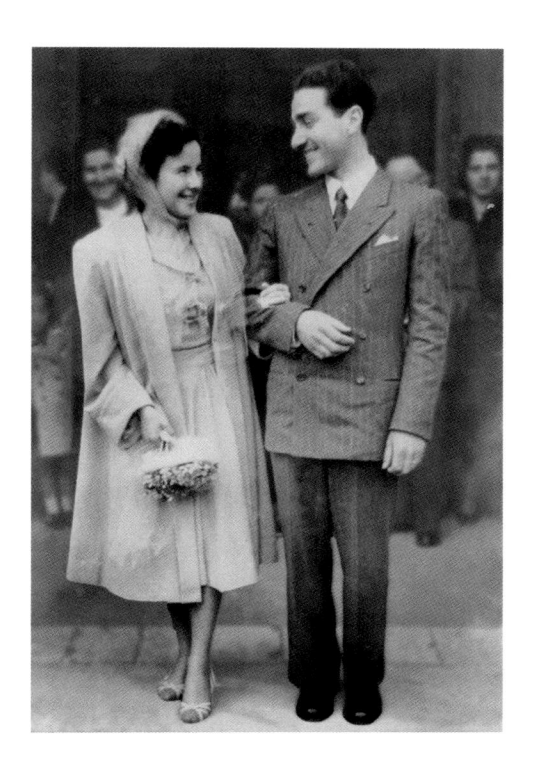

Mamma and papà's wedding, Rome, 5 April 1948

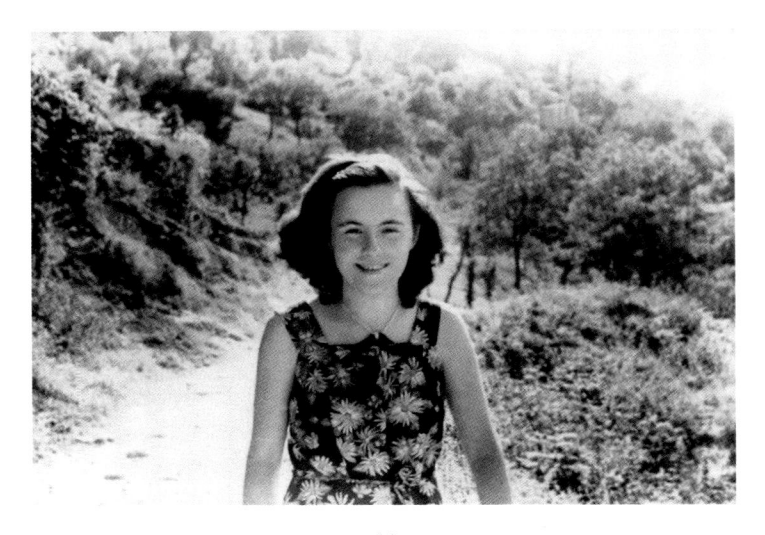

Mamma in Abbateggio, 1948

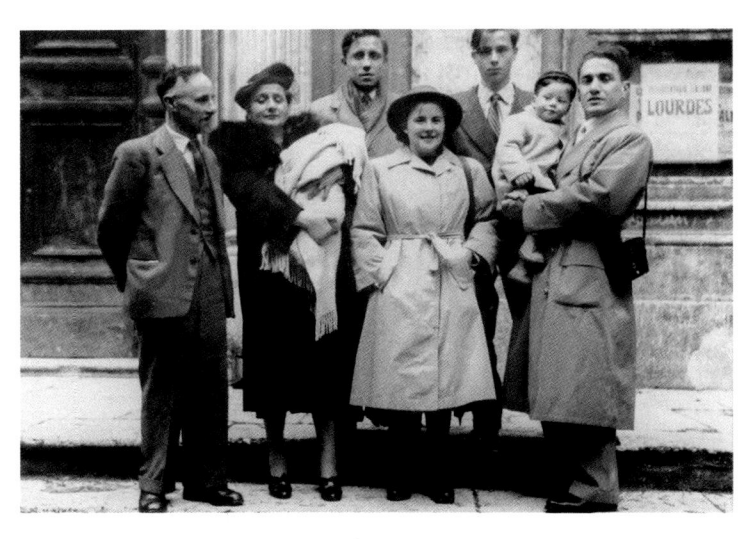

*Mamma, papà, Enrico and Silvia, with mamma's family,
departure for Tanganyika, March 1951*

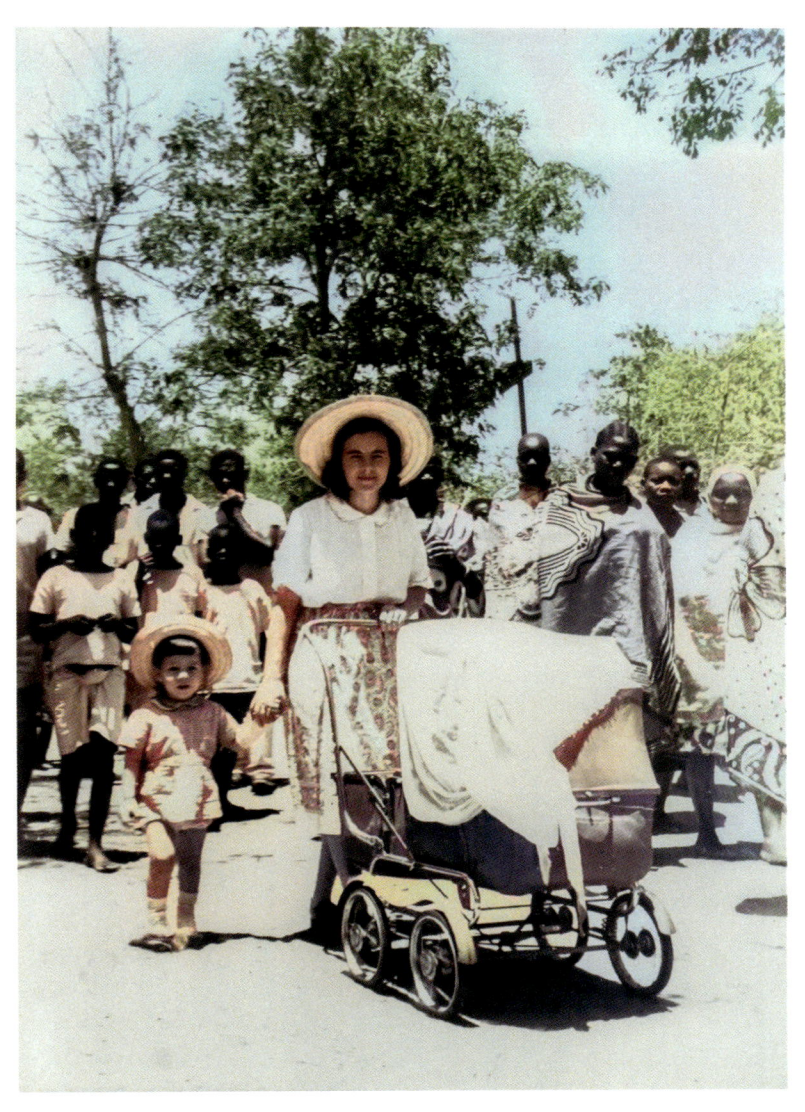

Mamma's arrival in Ukerewe, with Enrico and Silvia, 1951

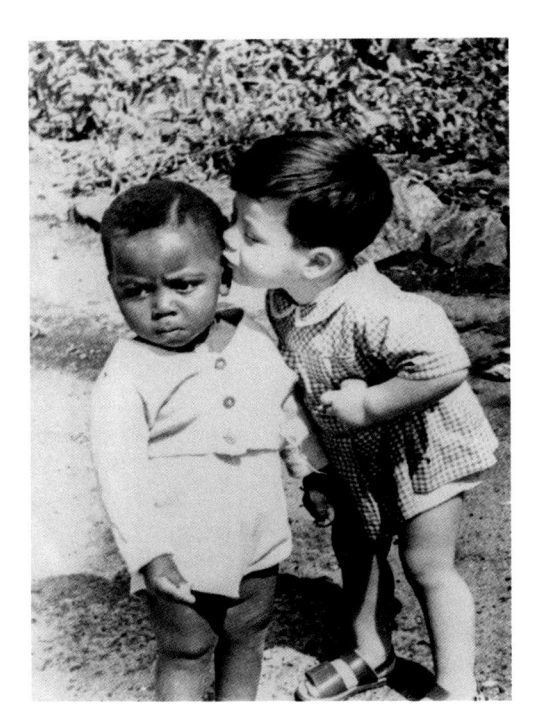

*Enrico and Francis,
Urambo, 1951*

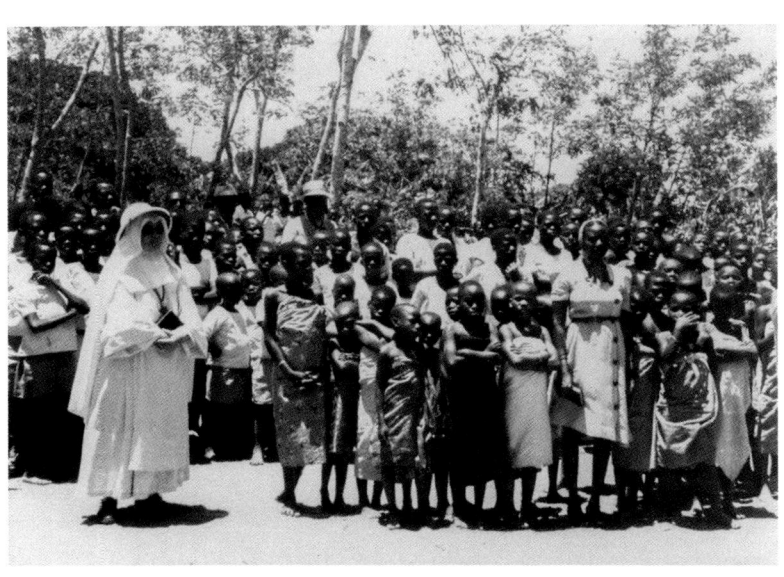

Mission schoolchildren with Sister Anne, Kagunguli, 1951

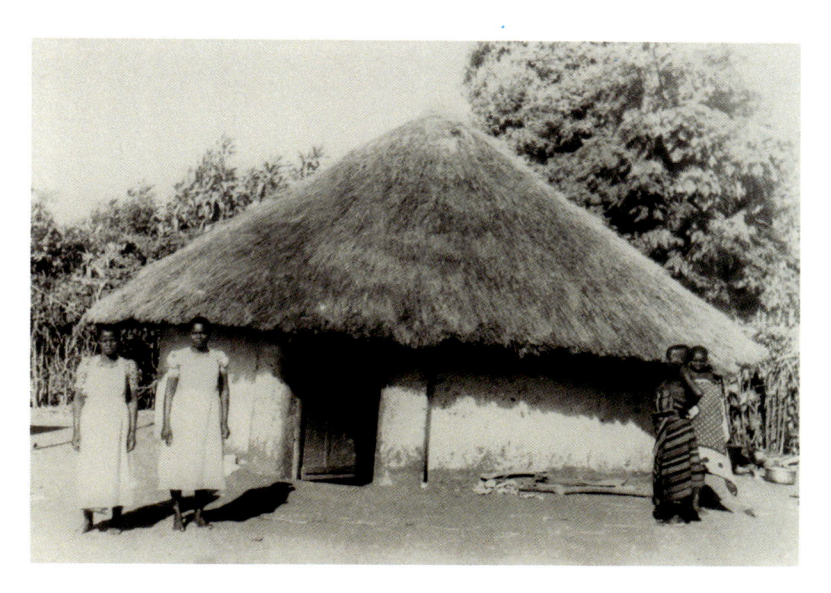

Old hospital 'ward', Kagunguli, 1951

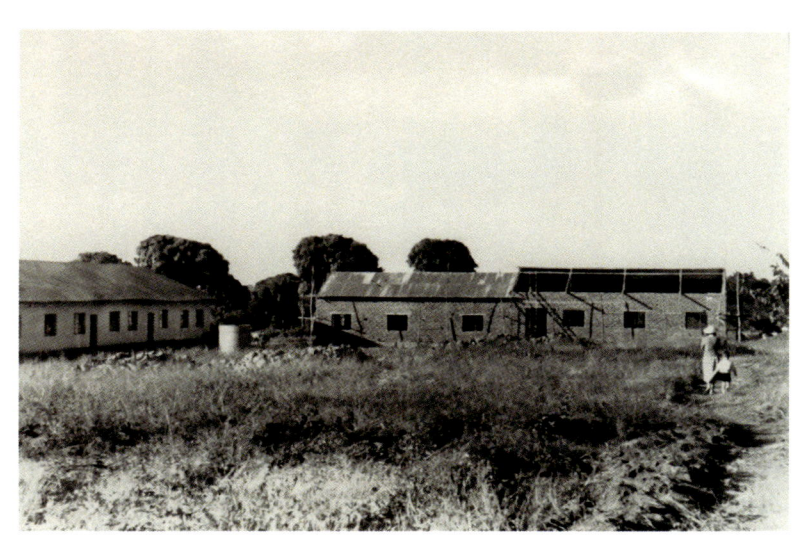

New hospital under construction, Kagunguli, 1952

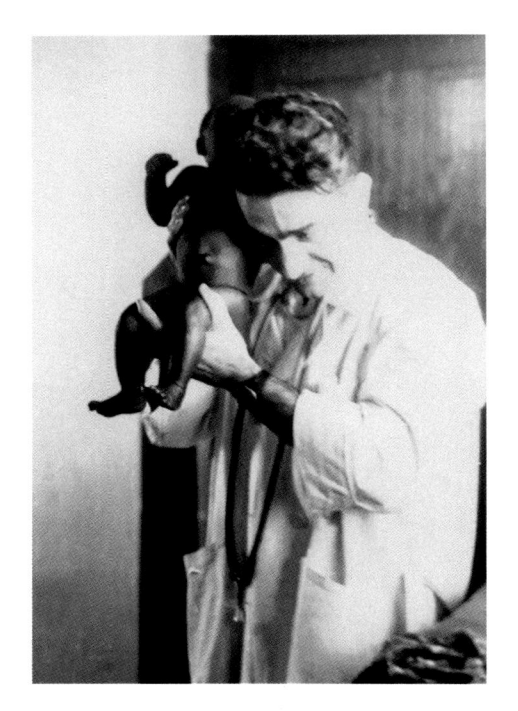

*Papà in the new hospital,
Kaguguli, 1952*

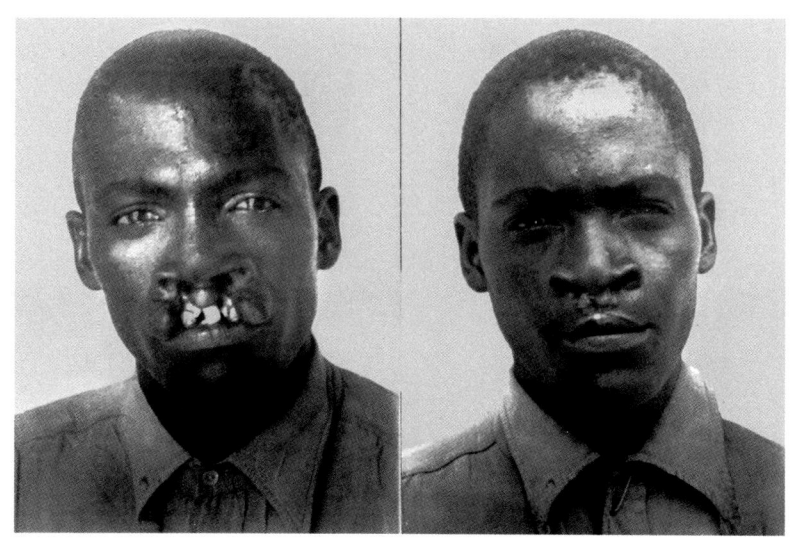

Cleft lip operation 'before' and 'after', Kagunguli, 1952

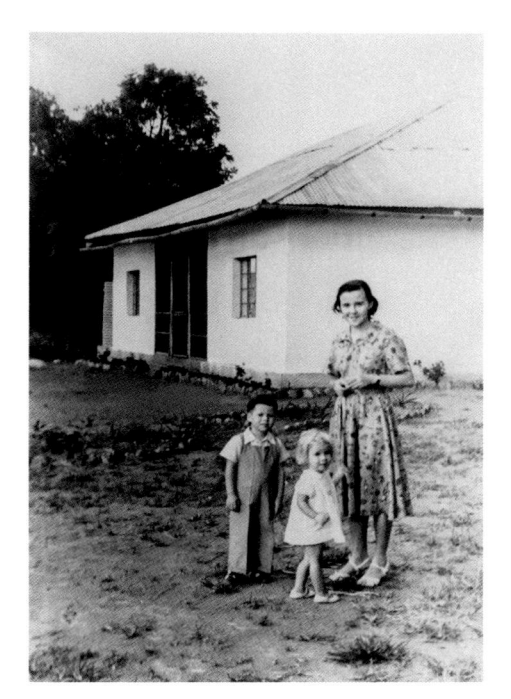

Mamma, Enrico and Silvia outside the new house in Kangunguli, 1952

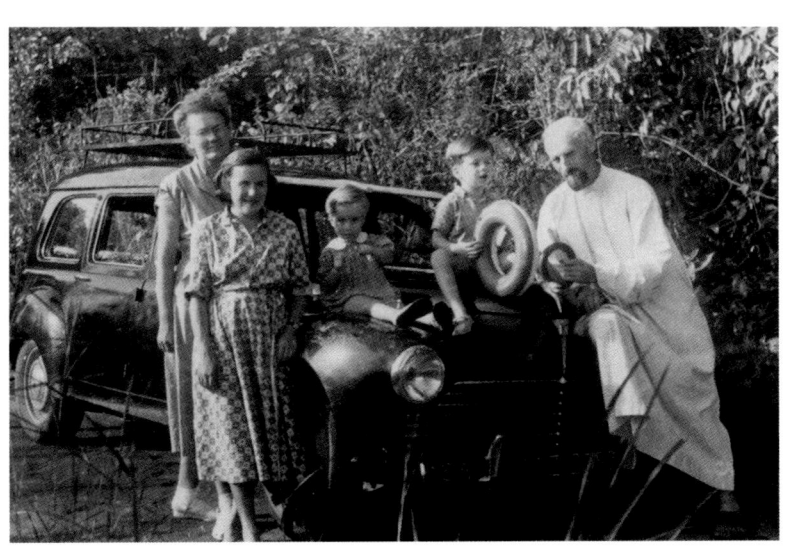

First Peugeot, lent by the Mission. Mamma, Silvia and Enrico, Dr Schroeder (a colleague from the mainland) and Fr van de Wee, 1953

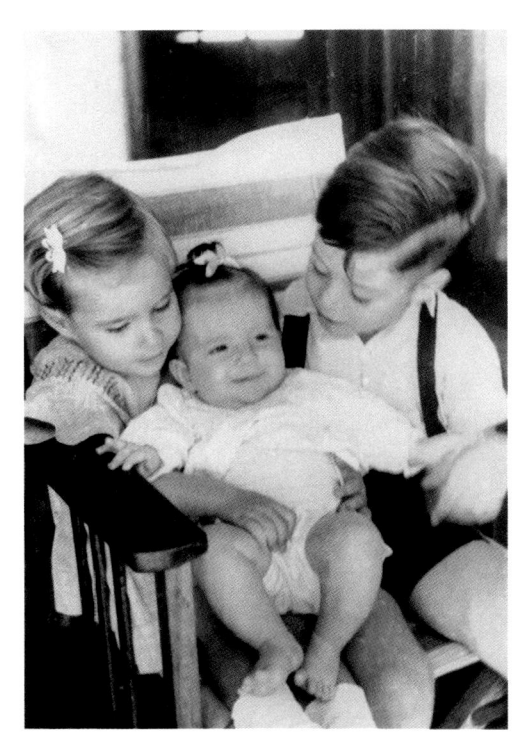

Enrico and Silvia with me, Kagunguli, June 1954

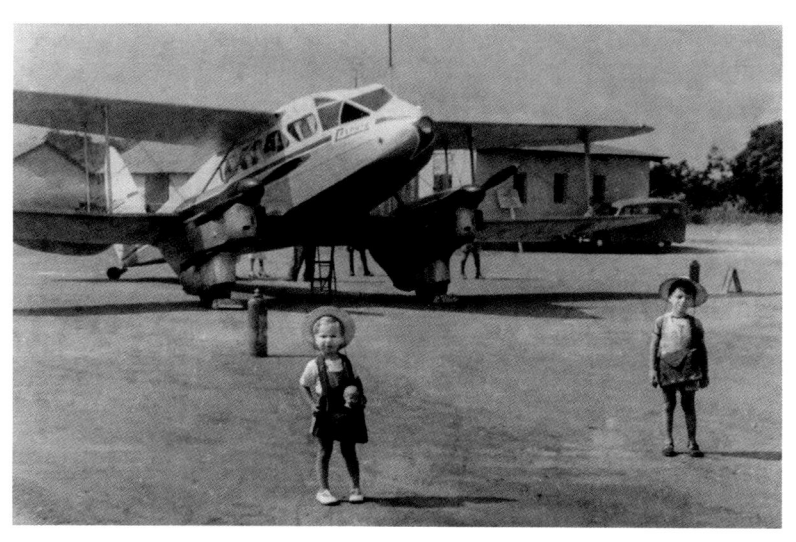

First leave to Italy, Mwanza airstrip, July 1954

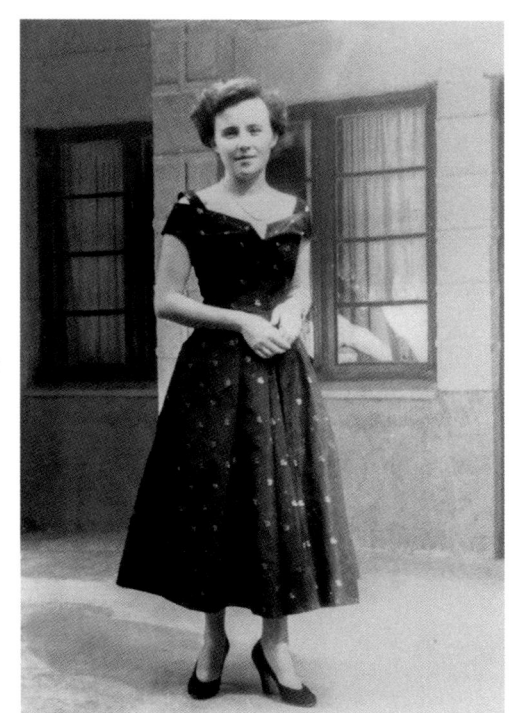

The Dress, Musoma, 1955

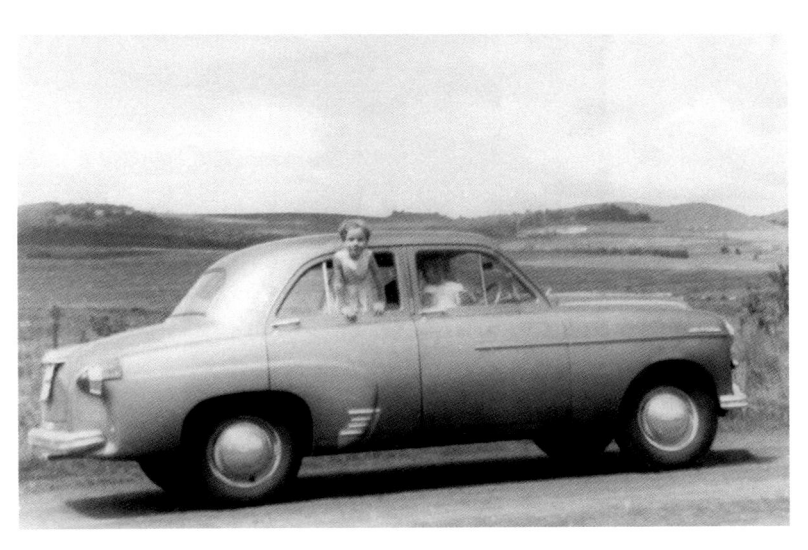

Silvia and me in our Vauxhall Wyvern, en route to Nairobi, 1956

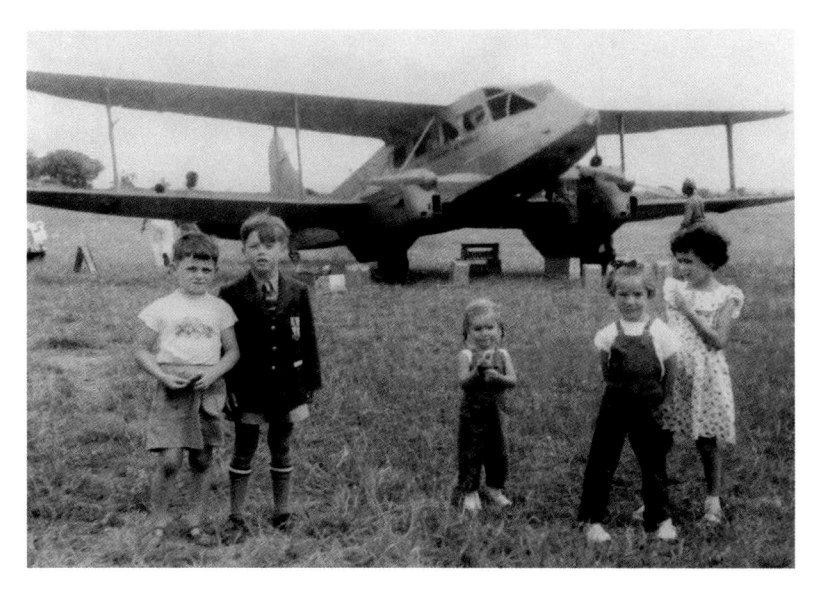

*Enrico travelling to school, Silvia and me in the middle,
and two friends, Musoma airstrip, 1957*

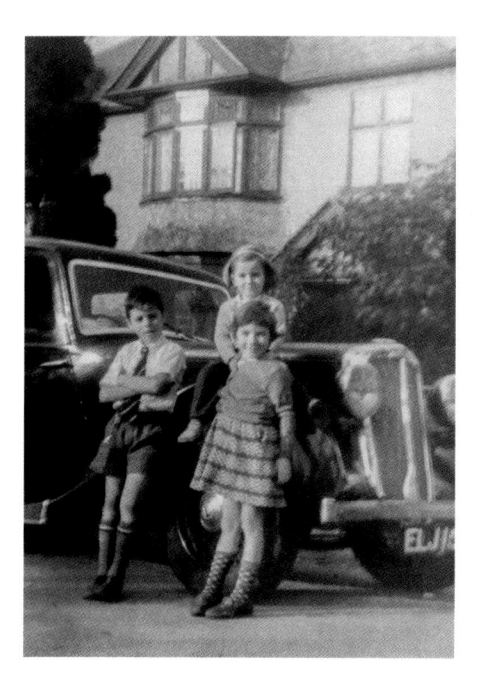

*Enrico, Silvia and me
with Miss Hancock's 1938
Lanchester 11, Bromley,
1958*

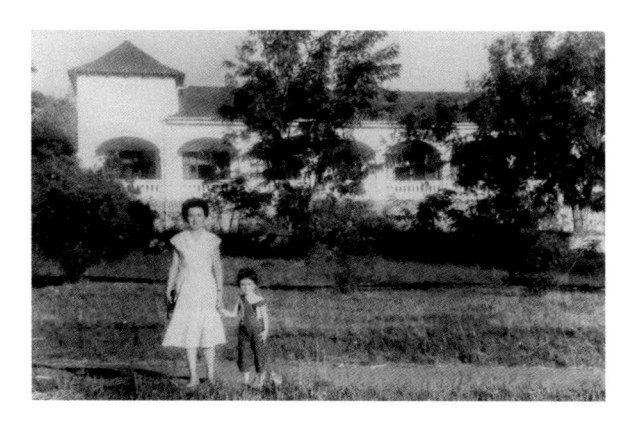

Mamma with me in front of the Kaiserhof Annexe, Kigoma, 1958

*The playhouse papà built,
Kigoma, 1958*

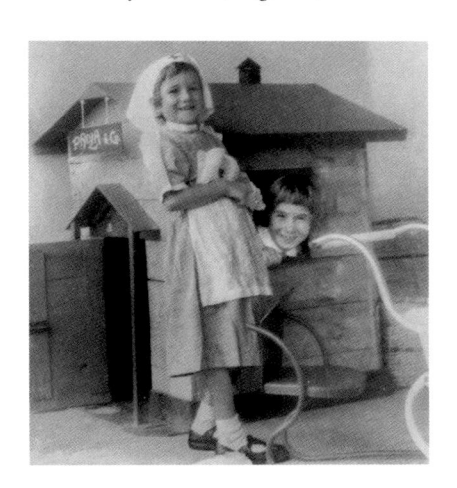

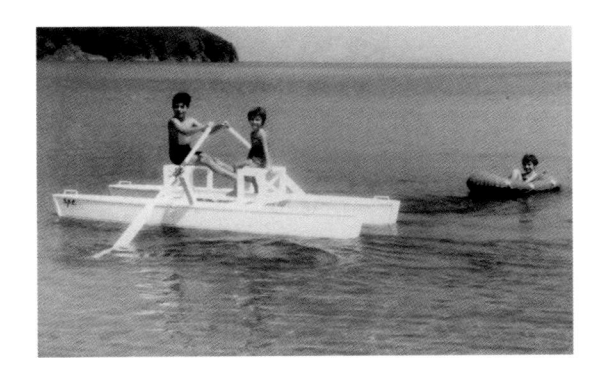

*The Spe,
Kigoma 1958*

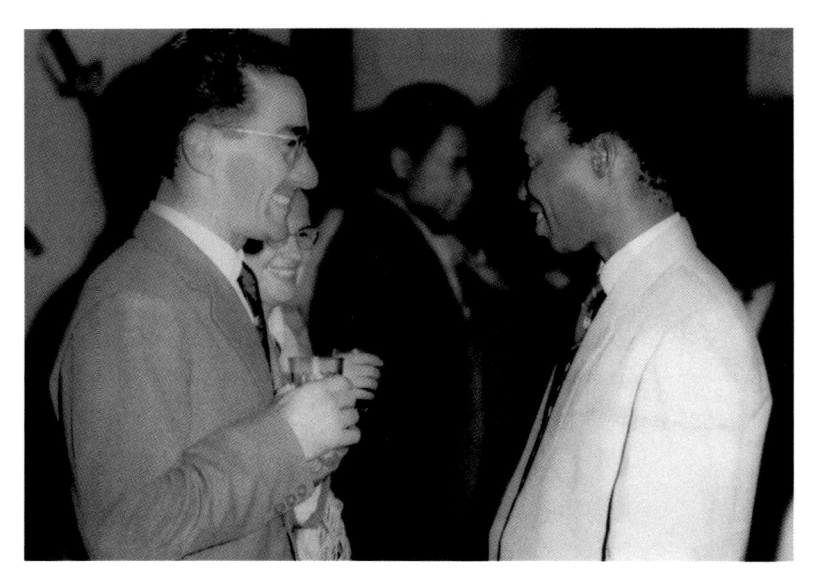

Papà and mamma with Mwalimu Julius Nyerere, Dar es Salaam, 1964

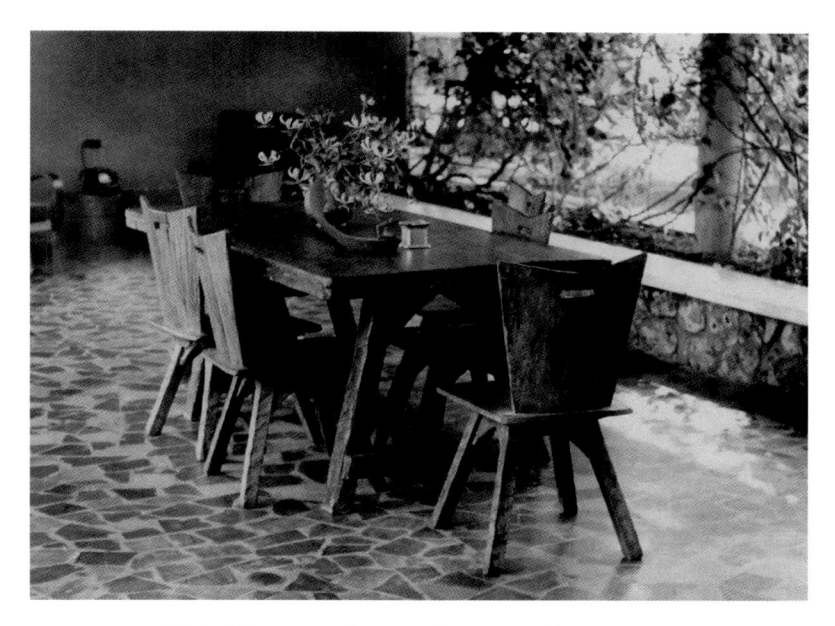

The Table, Kinondoni Road, Dar es Salaam, 1966

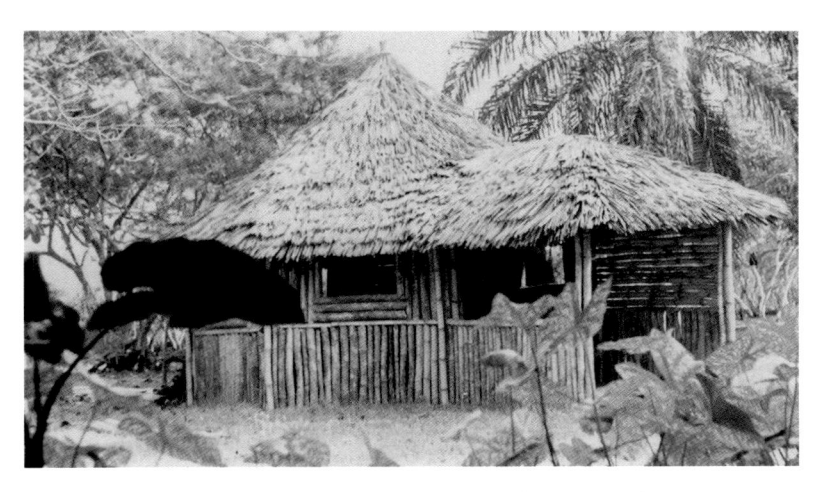

The banda my father built, Kinondoni Road, Dar es Salaam, 1966

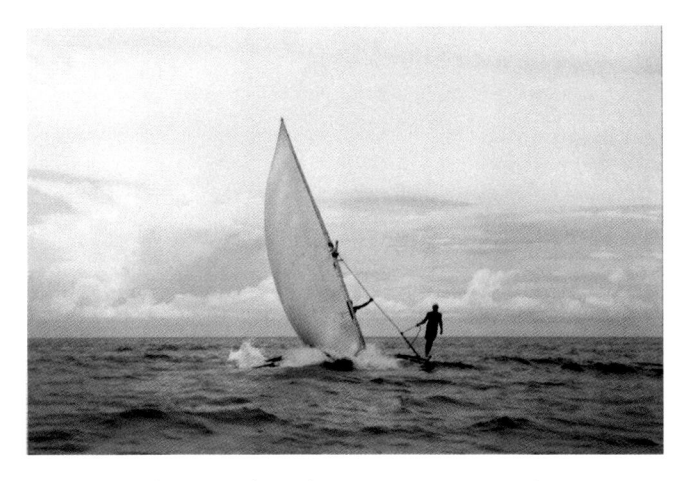

Ngalawa on the Indian Ocean, Dar es Salaam

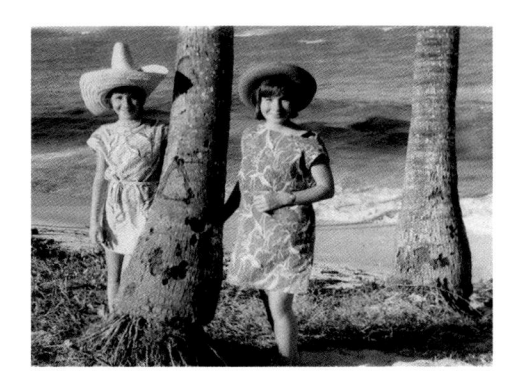

*Silvia and me, Oyster Bay,
Dar es Salaam, 1965*

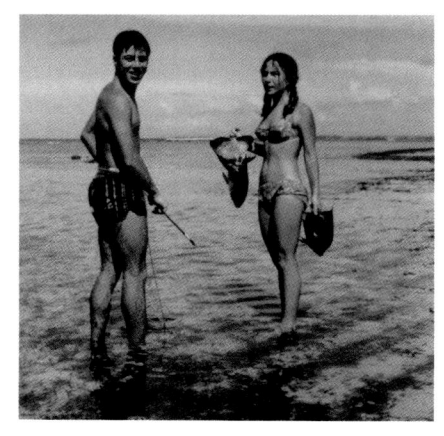

*Enrico and Silvia,
Dar es Salaam, 1968*

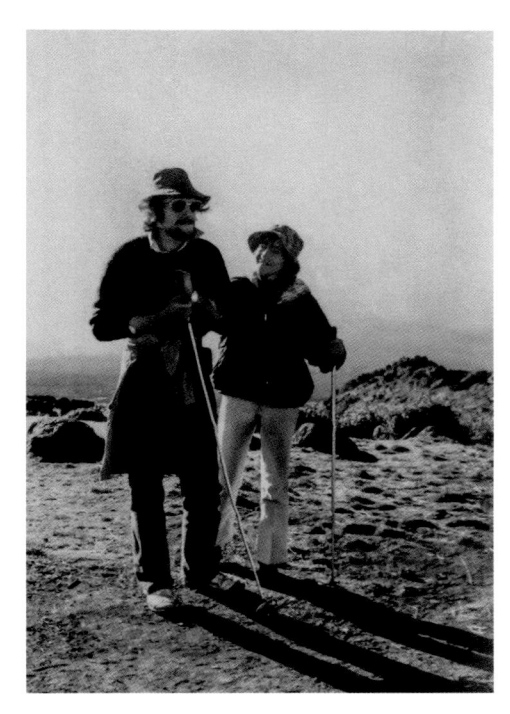

Willie and me at Gilman's Point, Kilimanjaro, 1974

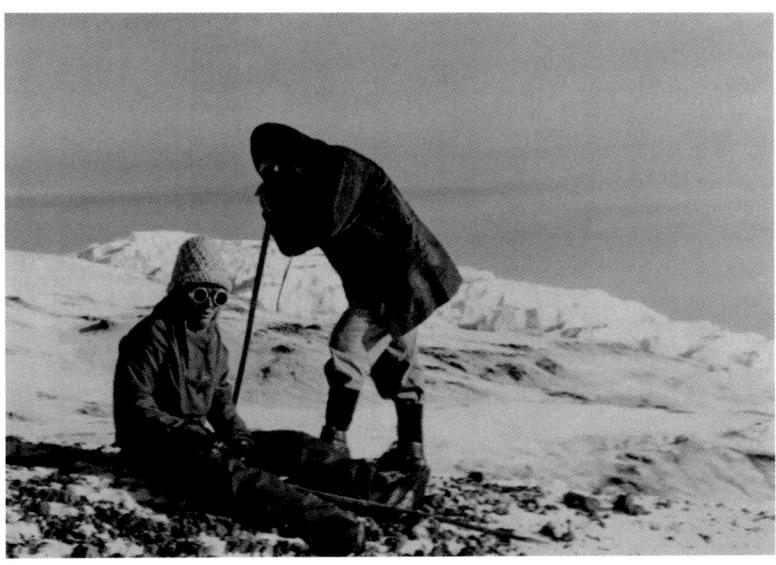

Christina (standing) and me at Uhuru Peak, Kilimanjaro, 1977

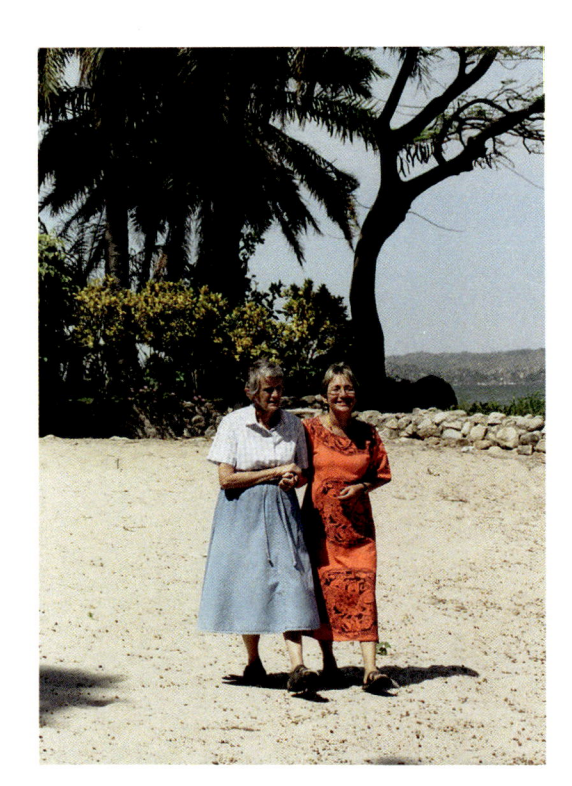

Sister Pauline and me, Mwanza, 2004

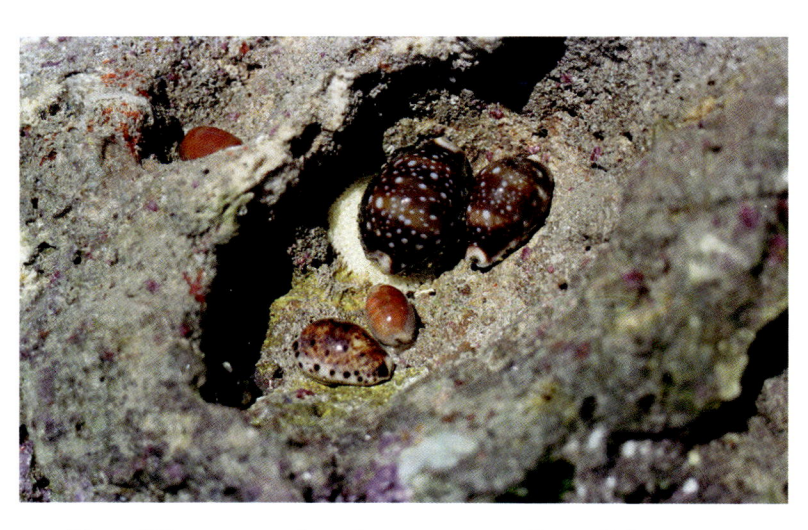

Three different types of cowries, one on eggs, Dar es Salaam, 2004

Crimson and Scarlet

At the beginning of term, Val and I scratched our wrists with a pin. I scrawled the letters KC for Keith Carrott. When both our wrists were bleeding, we pressed them tight against each other.

'We're blood sisters now,' Val said. 'For ever.'

But someone sneaked on us, and we were called to the Office. Heart thumping, bladder straining, I scratched over the letters. I didn't want any of the nuns to read them. And even more, I didn't want Silvia to see them. She would laugh and tell Enrico and I'd never hear the end of their teasing. By the time I reached the Office, my wrist was a mess of blood.

A nun – I don't remember who it was – stood there, nostrils flared, face beetroot, a ruler in her hand. Not a normal ruler, but one of the long board ones the teachers used.

'Show me.' Her voice was chillingly quiet.

I obeyed.

'And you, a doctor's daughter! Have you not heard of tetanus?' The second time in two terms that I'd been admonished with those words. This time they made sense.

'Put your hand out. No, palm down, not up.'

Thwack, thwack, thwack. Six strokes. I was shaking, my nose dripped, my eyes streamed, and my pants were wet. I didn't know which was worse, the pain or the shame. The back of my hand was as crimson as the blood on my wrist. *Crimson* became my least favourite word.

That term, Old Mother Florence – Flo –died of malaria. We filed past her open coffin in the Chapel. I'd never seen a dead person before. Her skin was white and waxy and made me think of Tomorrow blooms. Out near the sports fields were bushes with three colours of fragrant flowers. The dark purple ones were called Yesterday; the next day they would turn lavender and be called Today, and on the third day they were white: Tomorrow. After that they dropped off. We didn't have them in Mwanza. I thought it was a bit like being babies, growing up, getting old, and dying. Only we got longer than the flowers.

That evening we played 'Dare, Truth, Kiss, Command or Promise' after lights out. Val and I chose Dare. 'Dare you to go to the Chapel and stroke Flo's arm,' someone said. And we did, terrified that she'd come alive. She felt like cold rubber. We got away with it. I wonder how many *thwack*s it would have merited had we been caught.

A blood sister, the ruler and a death: enough for one term, I thought. At last, end of term came. But I didn't feel well.

Twenty uniformed girls stood by the Chapel at the Front of the House, as Michael, the driver, in his starched white uniform and cap, loaded our brown leather cases into the hold.

Silvia was chatting to her friends. My throat felt like sharp knives were cutting into it, and I couldn't wait to get home so that my father could make me better. The world started spinning around me. My legs were wobbly. I leaned on the bus and called Silvia.

'I feel dizzy,' I whispered.

'Listen, Titch, don't tell a soul, or they won't let you travel.' She gave me a hug. 'Your face is all hot and red.'

'I can't stand any more.'

'Go to the dorm and lie down. When the bus is ready to go, I'll come for you.' I slipped through the black wrought iron gate, into the Quad, up the stairs, along the verandah, and into my dormitory. All the beds had been stripped. On the wall by my bed was my Countdown Caterpillar, with his ten segments numbered backwards from his tail end, all crossed out, and the word *HOME* written across his head. I took off my shoes and blazer and lay down on the mattress.

My stomach lurched. I leaned over the side of the bed, and out it came, this morning's scrambled eggs and toast and tea, and the kedgeree and coconut custard we'd had for lunch, all in a smelly puddle over my patent leather Clarks. I wiped my mouth on my cardigan. My heart pumped and my cheeks were burning. My whole body ached. I opened the buttons on my blouse and saw them: red spots all over my stomach.

I heard a familiar clank. The heavy rosary beads the nuns wore around their waists always warned of their approach. You knew when Squirrel – Mother Cyril – was coming because she was inseparable from her dog, Ponky, who wore a bell around his neck. Which one would it be? Tickie? Minnie? I hoped it would be Minnie; she was kind. But what would she say about my sick on the floor? I threw my blazer over it.

Oh no… It was Sup who came in! Mother Superior herself! I had never spoken to her in my whole first two terms.

'Paola pet, what on earth has happened to you?'

'I want to go home,' I sobbed. 'I just want to go home.'

She put her hand on my forehead and told me to open my mouth. I was good at opening my mouth wide, because I hated the stick doctors used to put down throats. It made me gag.

'I'm calling Doctor Boyle right now.'

'But Silvia is waiting for me at the bus.'

'I'm sorry, pet; you're not going anywhere until you are better.

You just rest there a while, and we'll get you cleaned up, and make a bed. I'll call your parents.'

Not again! Last term I'd missed the train and boat safari because of measles, and now here I was once more...

Sup went away, and I fell asleep. I must have slept for hours. When I woke up, I was in my clean white nightie, in crisp sheets. Blubbery Doctor Boyle hovered over me with his stethoscope and cold hands. 'Scarlet fever,' he said, and gave me a huge pill that got stuck in my throat.

Scarlet. I had learnt that word from my colouring box, along with *vermilion* and *aquamarine* and *canary* and *crimson*. Crimson was the colour of blood. I shuddered as I looked at the scar on my wrist.

Perhaps this scarlet fever was a punishment for having been so naughty. But hadn't the ruler, plus Confession, which followed on the next Saturday, been enough?

I liked the word *scarlet*, but I didn't like *fever*. It made me feel I'd be sick for ever. My brain was too tired to think about words now, and I drifted off to sleep again. When I woke up it was the middle of the night. Sup was in a chair by my bed.

'I need the toilet,' I whispered, but I couldn't move.

Sup picked me up in her soft, wobbly arms and carried me to the end of the verandah. I remembered the time a few weeks before when a Big Girl had caught me washing my checked orange pyjama bottoms in the sink.

'What happened?' she'd asked.

'I left it too late,' I'd said, feeling my cheeks flush.

Back in bed I thought about Silvia and Enrico. They'd be chugging through the cold Rift Valley on the train now, sleeping under the scratchy grey blankets they'd rent for three shillings.

For days I drifted in and out of sleep, taking Doctor Boyle's medicines, and being carried to the toilet. I wondered whether Sup ever went to the toilet herself. I didn't feel hungry, but every now and then I had some soup or a scrambled egg. The other nuns came to visit me: Minnie brought me a soft rabbit, and a book called *Rhodesian Adventure*, but I was too tired to read.

Sup drew a new caterpillar for me, with lots of segments and no HOME at the end as she wasn't sure when I would be well enough to go.

I slowly got better and stronger. The spots faded, and on Day 6, Sup said, 'You're going home tomorrow… on the plane!' I was to travel with two Big Girls, Karen and Pat, from the nearby Kenya High School, which broke up for the holidays a week after us. The journey would take only two hours, instead of the two days it would have taken by train and boat.

Sup and Michael took me to the airport, where we met Karen and Pat. Both had long wavy hair tied in ponytails, Karen's dark, and Pat's blonde. They were sixteen. Double my age. Karen took me by the hand, and on the plane, I sat beside them, by the window. I was too scared to speak, and they chatted away, mostly about boys and makeup. They took out little compacts and applied mascara and scarlet lipstick.

The trip was bumpy, and I felt sick. As the plane approached Mwanza airport, we dipped below the clouds, and I looked through the window. I could see the lake, the Bismarck Rock, Capri Point where our house was, the Club and pool, and the runway. Two tiny figures were standing on the airstrip, looking up and waving. As we came closer, I could make out Enrico and Silvia. But they were knee deep in water.

'Due to weather conditions, we cannot land,' the pilot said. 'We will turn back to Musoma.' Musoma was two hundred kilometres away by road.

The rest of the journey is a blur in my mind. In Musoma, Karen, Pat and I stayed a night in a simple hotel room. How did we get there from the airport? Who paid for it? How were our parents informed of what was going on? That evening, Karen appeared from the bathroom with short hair, and explained that her long ponytail had been a *toupée*. I had never heard the word before.

The next morning, we set off on a fishing boat for Mwanza. I say 'fishing boat' because that is what I remember being told. I recall nothing about that part of the trip. I'm pretty sure it wasn't a luxury yacht… those did not exist in Musoma. Whose boat was it? How was it arranged? It must have had some sort of powerful engine, but even so, I imagine it took us all day to travel the distance. What did we eat? Who was with us? Were our parents worried? Oh, what I would give to find Karen and Pat and ask them if they remember the details… details more important than *toupées* and scarlet lipstick.

The Secret

Squidge, slosh, slide. We squealed as we trudged along the muddy riverbank in single file, our aprons straining at the waist as we pulled at each other's belts, tired and happy after an afternoon of play.

'Girls, you know the drill,' Frankie said as we approached the school grounds. Frankie was Mother Francis Michael: freckly and large with twinkly eyes, the kindest and most human of all the nuns. She wasn't on the teaching staff, because during the week she drove off to work in the biggest slum in Nairobi.

'Socks off,' Frankie said. We sat on the ground, and once we'd removed our shoes we wiped the mud off them with our socks, which we then tucked into our pockets. Frankie would get into trouble if Sup found out she'd allowed us to have such messy fun.

About twenty of us who lived too far to make the journey home for the long half-term weekend 'stayed in'. I'd watch mums and dads driving up the avenue to pick up their children who were leaping up and down in front of the Hall, but I wasn't envious. Because this was a time of treats. And it was safe.

At half-term the Big Girls and we Juniors were all mixed together, sharing three or four dorms. The food was much better than usual: we were given fresh toast for breakfast, rather than the term-time stale leftover bread that was sprinkled with water every day to keep it going. We had buns for tea, trifle for dessert, and even, on one occasion, strawberries and cream.

We strolled to nearby stables, where we could feed the horses. Many Loreto girls who lived in Kenya were from farms, and were used to horses, but to me these elegant animals were more exotic and intimidating than elephants or giraffes.

Sometimes we walked to a nearby Carmelite convent. Unlike our nuns – who taught us in the classroom, chatted to the priests from St. Mary's next door, hitched up their habits and ran around the hockey field coaching us, and occasionally sneaked us out of bounds on riverside rambles – the Carmelites devoted their lives to prayer and contemplation. Apart from a weekly visiting time, they were cut off from the world. Rumour had it that this was the only occasion when they were allowed to talk. We never saw them: they were hidden behind a curtain, speaking to us in whispers. I often wondered how prayer could be enough for them: didn't they miss their families, didn't they want the constant chatter of schoolchildren around them?

But I hadn't always remained at school for half-term. Boarders could go and stay with a friend if they had written permission from their parents. In my first term, Silvia and I went to an Italian family my parents knew, the Ballettos. Angela Balletto was in Silvia's class. Little did I know at the time – in fact I only learnt recently – that Angela's father, Giovanni, had been a prisoner of war in Nanyuki, about two hundred kilometres north of Nairobi. Bored with life in the camp, he and two fellow prisoners decided to climb Mount Kenya, which is over 5,000 metres high. In January 1943 they escaped, unarmed, with makeshift equipment, and attempted the ascent. Balletto and one of the others made it to the summit; the third man was too ill to go for the final peak. After eighteen days on the mountain, they broke back into their camp, and received a punishment of twenty-eight days in solitary confinement, which was reduced to seven for their heroism.

I could have put the weekend to much better use talking to Mr. Balletto about his escapade, rather than spending it moping around, bored because Silvia and Angela were good friends and so much older and more sophisticated than I was.

The next half-term, Silvia went to stay with a friend, Anne, who lived on a farm somewhere in the Rift Valley.

'I was eleven,' she remembers, 'and Anne's dad taught me how to drive their Land Rover. Imagine! We went out into the bush… that was the most exciting thing that's ever happened to me!'

She and Anne went out for a long walk by a river one day. 'We met a Maasai,' Silvia told me. 'He was a friend of Anne's. We chatted away, and when we were leaving, he took a double string of beads from around his neck and gave it to me. Look, I still have it.' She sniffs at it. 'It still smells of his sweat. Can you imagine a Maasai giving away one of his necklaces? I wonder if it was a proposition…'

I, too, was in the Rift Valley that half-term. A girl in my class, Carole, invited me to her farm. She was quiet, with thick auburn hair that reached halfway down her back, and sad, dark eyes. She was an only child. Her mother managed the farm, because her father was serving in the British Forces in Cyprus. Cyprus had become an independent republic in 1960, and the British kept bases there. I never understood why Carole's father was so far away rather than on his farm with his family.

Carole's mother was petite and pretty, with dark, curly hair. As she drove us down a long avenue to the farmhouse, I could smell roses in the cool, damp air. It felt like I imagined rural England to be, with neat hedges and barns and lawns represented by words our family never had any use for in the dry, arid places where we lived. Several local men who were sweeping and trimming stopped their work to greet us as the car pulled to a halt. Exhausted from the journey and the excitement, we flopped into bed after a light supper.

'We're going riding,' Carole said the next morning, after a copious breakfast of scrambled eggs on toast. I followed her to the stables, and she introduced me to the *sice* – the man who looked after their three horses. 'Here, you take Fupi,' she said to me, showing me the smallest one. *Fupi* means *short* in Swahili. 'I'll go with Rafiki.' *Rafiki* means *friend*. She taught me how to mount and dismount, and warned me never to stand behind the horse, never to startle it. She showed me how to pat its neck. And we were off. I was shaking, but managed to bump along. After a few minutes Carole promoted me to trotting, telling me to bob up and down in a way that seemed counter-intuitive, in disharmony with the horse's movement. I was glad when my lesson was over and I was on solid ground. 'I'll show you how I can canter and gallop,' Carole said, and charged off around the field.

That evening Carole's mother drove us for about half an hour down a rough track through trees to the Club in a nearby town. It was nothing like our Club in Mwanza: no pool, no films, and no children. Carole and I sat on a step watching the sun set behind the trees and sipping Cokes, while her mother lounged at the bar with about five European men. I don't remember seeing any other women there.

'She's drinking again,' Carole sighed. 'Vodka. I think it's because she misses Daddy.' Her mother was sipping from a long glass with clear liquid and ice in it. When she'd finished it, someone poured her another. We sat there for what seemed like hours, listening to the buzz of banter and laughter from the bar. At last Carole's mother stumbled out to call us. She slurred, 'Time to go home.' My hands were clammy as I squirmed into the back of the car. She stalled twice, and then we shot off into the forest at high speed.

'Mummy, slow down!' Carole screamed. 'You'll hit a tree! You'll kill us all!'

Trembling, I clung to Carole, and wondered whether Silvia was anywhere nearby. If we drove off into the trees and crashed, who would find us? Who would tell my parents? The journey seemed endless, but somehow, we made it back to the farm.

Carole and I never spoke about the incident, and we drifted apart. I didn't mention it to any classmates or nuns. It was only at the end of the next holidays that I plucked up the courage to tell my parents.

They were adamant. 'You and Silvia will never go out for half-term again.'

I felt a weight being lifted off my shoulders. I dreaded the thought of staying with strangers. It was a bit uncool to stay in for half-term, but at least it wasn't because I didn't have friends: I had a valid, secret reason.

Speedy Gonzales

In the Sixties, the coolest thing a Loreto Convent boarder could have was a St. Mary's brother who owned a pet snake. And if that snake was any colour other than green, you'd be the envy of the entire school.

One Sunday afternoon, at the beginning of a summer term, Enrico came over from Saints at visiting time. He led us to some bushes near the playing fields, where we could be out of sight of other visitors, pupils, and patrolling nuns.

'Look what I found, under a rock, by the river,' he whispered. And from his khaki shorts pocket he pulled out a snake. A glossy black one, about a foot long. 'He's a Cape Wolf. His name is Speedy Gonzales.' Pat Boone's single, 'Speedy Gonzales', was all the rage at the time. Silvia reached out her hands and Enrico let the snake slither onto her. I was hesitant, but stroked his head. I expected him to be slimy, but he was smooth and cool to the touch.

'Is he poisonous?' I asked.

'Semi-poisonous,' Enrico said. I wasn't overly reassured. 'He only poisons his prey.'

'And what's his prey?'

'Mostly baby lizards and chameleons, and ants and flies, but I haven't seen him eating anything yet.'

Enrico managed to keep Speedy G. hidden in a box for the whole term, letting him out for a slink around the dorm at night, and bringing him over to visit us on Sundays. His existence was top secret amongst Enrico and his friends: the only pets allowed at school were white mice and hamsters in cages.

At the end of term, Enrico smuggled Speedy G. onto the train. As the train puffed and steamed uphill into the Kenyan highlands, the reptile managed to escape from his box, sped out of the boys' compartment, and into Mother Germaine's.

Mother Germaine, our headmistress, was our escort on that trip, accompanying us overnight as far as the port of Kisumu. Escorts had been recently introduced, probably as a result of reports of schoolchildren's misconduct on previous trips. We loved Mother Germaine: she was a tough woman from County Tyrone, fair and straightforward. But folklore has it that Speedy G. was too much for Mother Germaine's nerves. She leapt onto her bunk and screamed, and when Enrico came in and retrieved his reptile, she locked the door and wasn't seen again for the rest of journey.

In Kisumu, we had to put in a day before catching the overnight steamer around the lake to Mwanza, so, as usual, we strolled off to a White Fathers' mission where we were offered lunch by the priests. Speedy G. behaved impeccably and wasn't noticed.

When we docked into Mwanza port the next day, my mother met us in our VW Beetle. She was always so excited to see us. And this time, at last, I'd managed not to fall ill at the end of term, so we were all together from the start.

'Kids, we're going to have such fun! You've all had good reports, and you can just relax, and do anything you like…'

'Anything we like?' Enrico asked. 'How would you feel about a pet snake?'

'No problem.' My mother laughed.

Enrico fished in his shorts pocket. 'Mamma, meet Speedy Gonzales.'

The car swerved and my mother jammed on the brakes.

After a few days she got used to him. Enrico and Silvia had developed a new way of carrying him around, and you could tell where he was: whichever of them had their T-shirt tucked into their shorts had him around their middle. I, being The Titch, was not allowed to handle him on a regular basis. Nor did I want to.

In the evenings, when all the mums and small kids had gone home from an afternoon at the pool, we would traipse down the sandy track to the Mwanza Club, and Speedy G. would have his evening swim, doing lengths between Enrico and Silvia to the strains of Brian Hyland's 'Ginny Come Lately' and Neil Sedaka's 'Breaking Up is Hard to Do' crackling from the ancient loudspeakers at the poolside. In the water Speedy Gonzales seemed to me to writhe in time to the music.

'Snakes are deaf, Titch,' Enrico said. 'They don't have ears.'

'Maybe, but I bet they can feel the vibrations,' I said.

There was something that worried us about Speedy Gonzales: he didn't have an appetite – we never saw him eat. We offered him dead flies, live flies, mosquitoes, even once a scorpion we found in the pool. We encouraged him with lizards and geckos, but his jaws remained firmly shut.

Enrico knew all about Cape Wolves. 'They can survive ninety-nine days without food,' he told us. 'Speedy G. isn't even flicking his tongue in the air. That's how they sense that there's food around. He must be depressed.' As the days went by, we hunted for insects and small reptiles, cajoled him, stroked his back, but to no avail.

We decided that maybe it was being in captivity that had traumatised him. So on Day Ninety-Nine, the three of us went down to the bottom of the piece of dry scrubland we called our garden, and with tears in our eyes, we released him.

EDINBURGH

1963-1964

Spaghetti's the Only Veg

'You must be the new Italian girl from Africa. Close the door. We don't have servants here to close doors after us…'

This was my welcome to St. Margaret's Convent in August 1963, when our family moved to Edinburgh for nine months. My father, sponsored by the British administration in Tanganyika, was to study for a Diploma in Public Health. I was nine, Silvia twelve, and Enrico fourteen.

I shot back to close the door and looked over the bowed heads of thirty girls writing at their desks, towards the small, surly nun who had spoken to me. Mother Ignatius.

I could just about decipher her tight vowels. I wanted to yell that servants didn't close doors for us at home in Tanganyika because it was hot, unlike Edinburgh, and we left doors open so that we could get a bit of air. But I didn't say anything, because I was scared, and my accent was different, and I didn't want to stand out.

I was an outsider. 'New'. 'Italian'. 'From Africa'. 'Has servants'. Those were the labels branded on my forehead. And as soon as I opened my mouth, another was added. 'Posh'.

What hurt me the most about the servants quip was that it was true. In Tanganyika we did have house staff: a houseboy who cooked and cleaned, and a *shamba* boy who spent his days vainly attempting to tidy the scrub that surrounded our house, and to grow an occasional flower or a few vegetables here and there. When we were small, we had an *ayah* who looked after us and carried us on her back in a brightly-coloured cloth called a *kanga*. But Mother Ignatius' tone was all wrong. She didn't understand. These people called my mother *Mama* and my father *Daktari*. They lived with their families in a bungalow on our premises. My father delivered their babies, and attended to them when they were sick. We played with their children. That was the way it was for European families in that place at that time. And whenever we left one town for another, we cried, and they cried.

At school in Nairobi there were people to help run the place: Matthias the cook, waiters, several male cleaners, the *dhobi* and his assistants who washed our clothes, groundsmen, and *askaris* who patrolled the grounds at night to fend off trespassers. They lived 'out of bounds' in a little settlement behind the tennis courts and had a *duka* that supplied all manner of groceries. We would sneak out there to buy Black Cat bubble gum… and the Big Girls bought cigarettes. A mutual understanding ensured that the local staff never split on us.

Compared with Nairobi, Edinburgh was lacking in colour and fresh air. Although annual rainfall wasn't much higher, it was a constant drizzle spread evenly throughout the days, weeks and months. In Nairobi, rain was confined to two rainy seasons. By the end of the dry seasons, our skins were flaky, and our throats parched. We would draw pictures of the sun on the murram netball court and stamp on them day after day, until at last the angry clouds gathered, thick as dreadlocks, and burst open, unleashing their loads that crashed onto the roofs and fields.

But in some ways, St. Margaret's wasn't that different from Loreto. Academically we slotted in and did well. People looked after the place: gardeners and cleaners and kitchen staff; only here they were Scottish rather than Kenyan. The dinner ladies were kind and called us *hen*. We lined up for lunch in the refectory. Three deep vats were set out on a counter: one with meat, one with potatoes, and one with vegetables. We had to say 'little', 'lot', or 'nothing' for each one, so if we wanted lots of meat and potatoes and not much veg, we'd say 'lot, lot, little'. Just the smell of the food made my stomach churn and my palms sweat: tasteless grey meatballs, rissoles, sausages, and haggis were all variations of each other, generally accompanied by khaki cabbage floating in slimy liquid, and hemispheres of old mashed potatoes. I usually said 'nothing, nothing, nothing.' One day the dinner lady said to me, 'Spaghetti's the only veg today, hen.' I began to salivate but discovered that 'spaghetti' meant tinned hoop-shaped noodles in a sweet tomato sauce. Already skinny ('Chickenlegs' was among Enrico and Silvia's many nicknames for me), I quickly started losing weight. My parents were worried, so I was taken off school dinners. Every day my father would leave the university to take me out to lunch, so he could check that I was eating properly. Great for me, but I think it wasn't much fun for him.

Silvia settled well, and soon picked up an Edinburgh accent. I wished I had one too, but it didn't happen.

Enrico went to a school called Scotus Academy.

'We used Murrayfield Stadium for our rugby matches,' he remembers. 'It was next door. I used to play barefoot, and everyone was shocked.'

'Didn't you have rugby boots?'

'Of course I did, but at Saints it was cool to play barefoot, and I figured it would be even cooler in Edinburgh.'

Enrico also remembers that at Scotus Academy, punishment was a leather belt on the palm, rather than a cane on the backside. 'It hurt a lot more.'

'What did you get belted for?'

'Same as Saints... missing prayers, stockings not hitched up properly...'

We had swapped houses with a doctor who went off to Tanganyika to do my father's job while we were away. His semi-detached house was in the village of Currie, some twelve kilometres southwest of Edinburgh. Dull suburbia.

My father drove us in to school, and we'd get the bus back in the afternoon, stopping to spend our pocket money on sweets on the way: sherbet with a liquorice straw, flying saucers, love hearts with messages like *Only You* stamped on them, Liquorice All Sorts, fruit gums, fruit pastilles, gobstoppers... there was no end to the variety.

Back home, we'd quickly do our homework, then park ourselves on the carpeted floor in front of the TV. Screen time had no limit. We had never had a TV before, and we would watch everything from *Z Cars* and *The Saint* to *Bonanza* and *The Lone Ranger* to wrestling and snooker. I learnt to recognise double nelsons and cinch positions. We watched *Juke Box Jury* and *Ready, Steady, Go*, and practised saying, 'It's got a good beat' in Scots accents with all the correct glottal stops. We witnessed the rise of Beatlemania, the fanatic movement that gripped the U.K. and the world, and watched our screens, gobsmacked, while mobs of adulating young girls screamed uncontrollably as they followed the band around on their tours. But we remained faithful Rolling Stones fans: as with Elvis and Cliff (Enrico carefully greased back his Elvis quiff and groomed his ducktail), you couldn't be both.

My father was in heaven: he loved studying, but I wonder how my mother felt. She never complained, but I remember she was always cold. The first time she hung the washing out on the line in the back garden, the neighbour, Mrs. Smith, rang the doorbell. 'We don't hang underwear outside in this neighbourhood, Maria,' she scolded. My mother had a whole new culture to absorb.

When it came to the summer term, we were supposed to change into summer uniforms, but my mother refused to buy them for us. 'It's freezing cold here,' she said. 'Why should we spend money buying clothes that are completely unsuitable for the climate, just for a few weeks?' So, with burning cheeks, I would sink into my itchy tunic, while all around me my classmates blossomed in their fresh checked cotton frocks.

My mother was right; it wasn't for long. Soon it was time to return to Africa. While we were in Scotland, there had been huge political changes: following the Sultanate of Zanzibar's independence in 1963, the Zanzibar Revolution broke out in early 1964. The Sultan was overthrown, and thousands of Arab Zanzibaris were massacred. In April a union was formed between Tanganyika and Zanzibar, and the new nation of Tanzania was born.

Over the years we had worked our way from the village of Kagunguli on Ukerewe Island through increasingly larger towns: Musoma, Kigoma, and Mwanza. Now we were headed to Dar es Salaam, the capital, on the Indian Ocean coast. At last, we were to live in a real city: a city by the beach.

My father looked forward to putting his new knowledge into practice, my mother was always happy to go along with whatever made him happy, and we three craved the lifestyle that was familiar to us: sunshine, bare feet, and open spaces. Little did I know then how important those nine months in Edinburgh would be to me in determining my path in later years.

DAR ES SALAAM AND NAIROBI

1964-1966

Haven of Peace

Vendors selling ivory and ebony carvings at street corners; pokey incense-scented Indian *duka*s overflowing with fabrics, ribbons, zips, and buttons; multi-storeyed hotels, the like of which we had never seen; an air-conditioned – yes, air-conditioned – supermarket where, in its clinically scrubbed aisles, you could find a new-fangled curdy substance called *yoghurt* in glass jars, almost palatable if you laced it with plenty of sugar; a constant humid breeze heavy with the smell of seaweed and sewage wafting in from the ocean, gluing our cotton shirts to our bodies; humming markets displaying heaps of mangoes, pawpaws, and pineapples – the aroma of rotting fruit mingled with marijuana used to make Silvia high, she remembers; Dar es Salaam – the name means Haven of Peace – was a shock to our senses.

We arrived in August 1964. Dar, as we came to know our home town, had a population of over 200,000: ten times more than that of Mwanza, our previous Tanganyikan post.

This meant opportunities: my mother found paid work for the first time in her life, as an occasional interpreter/translator for visiting Italian and French business people. She soon taught herself to type and got a job with an Italian company, Snamprogetti, who were building an oil refinery on the far side of the port. As well as making an important contribution to the household income, she was delighted to have a newly found freedom, and to be able to use her skills outside the home.

My father worked in the outpatients' department at the Ocean Road Government Hospital, surrounded by a team of qualified colleagues and up-to-date equipment.

He was a great admirer of President Mwalimu Julius Nyerere, whose children would go to consult him barefoot, wearing tattered shorts and T-shirts. After graduating from Edinburgh University, where he had been one of only two black students from East Africa, Nyerere had worked as a schoolteacher in Musoma, which is where my father had first met him. Later, Nyerere was an anti-colonial political activist, and became the country's first president in 1962.

On Sundays we attended Mass at St. Peter's Church, a modern sparkling white building whose structure was entirely lattice-worked in stone, which made it bright and breezy. We often saw Nyerere there, with his wife and seven children.

Our social life was transformed. My mother's cousin Vari and his wife Marta now lived in Dar, and with family nearby, my mother had support. Never before in Africa had we seen so many Europeans. There was no TV, but we had plenty of entertainment. The Italian community numbered well over three hundred, and a small Italian Club showed films, served reasonably good food, and had tombola every Friday evening. The British community patronised the old colonial-style Gymkhana Club, which had an arid golf course and several tennis courts.

Dar had about six or seven cinemas, including a brand new drive-in, and my father loved taking us to watch whatever was showing: westerns, war films, crime thrillers, and his favourite genre, spy thrillers. Often he would watch the same film two or three times, to check that he hadn't missed anything.

Unlike the other places in Tanganyika where we had lived, Dar was swelteringly hot and humid all year round. What we loved most was the ocean. Our first house – a standard government bungalow with all the same Public Works Department furniture we'd had in previous posts – was in Lincoln Road, at one end of the palm-fringed mile-long Oyster Bay. Just before dawn broke each morning, streaking the sky with orange and red over the ocean, my father woke with the birds. Often he would turn on his reel-to-reel tape recorder to preserve the magic of the dawn chorus. He loved the variegated melodies, but took no interest in the bird species: it was only years later that we learnt to identify the robin chat's urgent plea gradually fading like a marble bouncing down a stone stairway, and the tapping crescendo of the kingfisher welcoming the day. When the concert was over, he would jog the length of the beach and back, dragging along whichever of us children was willing to accompany him. I often went, but was too lazy to jog with him.

'If you can complete the two miles in under sixteen minutes,' my father would say, 'you are fit.' He always did. Not bad, on a soft sand track.

I had a dog called Nerone, a Labrador cross, at the time. He loved coming to the beach. As my father jogged, I would lie in the sand, which was still cool from the night, while Nerone went wild, sniffing at crabholes, and digging fast and deep until at last he caught the hapless inhabitant in his jaws, shook its last breaths out of its being, tossed it aside, and moved on to sniff at the next hole.

At high tide, the sandy north end of Oyster Bay, where we lived, was best for swimming, with great waves for body surfing. At low tide, the coral reef at the south end, which extended close to the beach, would be exposed. There we could swim in rock pools, brave it to the breakers pounding and frothing beyond the reef, or walk on the hardened coral, examining starfish, brittle stars, and multi-coloured sea urchins. Tripping onto sea urchins was not much fun: their spines were poisonous, and the puncture wounds often became infected. Our immediate remedy was to dab the area with urine, then apply pawpaw, which was supposed to soften the spines, and suck them out.

During the rainy seasons, we had to take care, as blubbery jellyfish filled the waters near the shore and were often washed up on the beach. More dangerous for its fierce sting was the jellyfish's relative, the spindly purple-tinged Portuguese man o' war. The pain inflicted from brushing a tendril was excruciating.

A favourite game was to pick up a sea cucumber and chase each other, squeezing it tight till its liquid squirted out.

After only a few months in Lincoln Road, we moved to a house that became vacant in Garden Avenue, a street lined with flamboyant trees, close to the hospital. When we arrived, we found a birdbath in the acacia-shaded garden. It was a giant clam shell – sixty or seventy centimetres across – perched atop a metre-high, ancient, fossilised tree trunk. Silvia was fascinated by it.

The house was German-built, similar to the one we'd occupied in Capri Point in Mwanza, with two central rooms surrounded by verandahs, netted off to make more rooms. Silvia and I, as always, shared a bedroom. Towards the end of the Garden Avenue phase, Silvia improvised a curtain, which she hung across the room, so we at last had a semblance of our own spaces. Over the years she developed her sewing skills, and one of our favourite trips was to the Indian quarter where we would shop for fabrics and trimmings, along with Simplicity and Butterick patterns, which she would use to fashion complicated dresses, hats, and shorts. I was delighted to be her sidekick, and learnt all sorts of new words, like *tacking* and *facings* and *bias binding*. I once left a pair of dressmaking scissors open on a sisal mat, and she still has the resulting scar.

Shortly after we arrived in Dar, our recently widowed paternal grandmother, Nonna Maria, came to visit. Her trip was such a success that two years later she returned with our maternal grandmother, Nonna Vittoria. We found it incredible that women of their advanced years would undertake such an arduous trip. They were in their mid-sixties. They enjoyed the beach, loved cooking, and simply slotted in as part of the family. We took them to Mikumi National Park where they were amazed by the wildlife, and on a day trip to visit Bagamoyo, a town sixty kilometres along a rough sandy track up the coast.

In the late nineteenth century, Bagamoyo was the first capital of German East Africa. It had been a trading centre for fish and salt from the thirteenth century. By the eighteenth century it was the largest trading port along the east central coast of Africa, and a century later, it developed into a prosperous market for slaves and ivory. This is when it acquired its name (originally Bwaga-Moyo), which means 'leave down your heart' in Swahili, and is sometimes interpreted as meaning 'give up all hope'. Despite its tragic history, as I wandered around ancient ruins of tombs and mosques, spotting the occasional grazing goat or scuttling hen, with the sound of the ocean waves in the background, I felt a sense of immense peace. Bagamoyo was an antidote to the hustle and bustle of Dar.

In those early Dar days, Enrico and Silvia had a new nickname for me: 'Stinker'. It originated from my mother's affectionate (so she thought) pet name she had given me when I was a baby: 'Pussetti', a corruption of the Italian word for 'smelly'. Stinker was meant as lighthearted fun, and I tried to be stoical about it, but occasionally my eyes would well up with tears. One day my mother asked, 'What's the matter?' and I told her. A family council was called, and my father explained that this sort of teasing could be hurtful.

'What would you like to be called?' Enrico asked. 'Let her have whatever name she wants.'

'Killer,' I said. 'From now on, my name is Killer.'

Silvia and Enrico embraced the new nickname, in a teasing sort of way. It was confirmed on the sign on the tree where my father built us a treehouse: Killer's Den. I was now the proud owner of a dog, a treehouse, and a great name that stuck for a couple of years.

Our Garden Avenue house was just a couple of hundred metres from the beachfront at Ocean Road: less pleasant than Oyster Bay. A large sewage pipe led out to sea, and at low tide the stink was overpowering.

The Hindus had a crematorium along Ocean Road, and Silvia had a friend, Claretta, who lived in an apartment near there. Whenever anyone heard the fires being lit, they would yell 'Bombay Grill!' and everyone would close their windows.

On Sunday evenings the Indian community would drive their cars in convoy along Ocean Road, ('Exactly 22 m.p.h.,' we would joke, and strangely enough, that was indeed their speed) looking for a place to park and look out to sea. We imagined they were paying homage to Gujarat, the home their ancestors had left a century before. 'They live in cramped conditions,' my mother would say. 'They need to get some air.' I wince when I remember that we used to call their Sunday drive 'the Bombay Crawl', but it wasn't meant spitefully. The European, Asian and African communities lived side by side peaceably, if separately.

Dar had a brand new International School, but it seemed logical for us to continue attending our familiar schools in Nairobi. Economically, things were looking up for the family, so we were able to travel to school by plane – a journey of just an hour or two, depending on whether the plane stopped en route or not. Gone were the adventure school voyages that lasted several days.

Life felt stable. After years of moving house every couple of years, always to a town a bit larger than the last, we had arrived in the capital. There was nowhere better we could aspire to. We were here to stay. Perhaps this would become a definitive 'home'.

Back in Nairobi, a lot of changes had taken place in the year that we had missed while in Edinburgh.

Playing the Part

'You're a newbug.' *Newbug*. That was almost as offensive as *daybug*. The girl who addressed me – Ella – had long, blonde hair, lank and greasy. Me? New? It was she who was the newbug. I'd just been away in Scotland for a few months. This had been my school long before it was hers, but I felt like an alien.

We now had curtained-off cubicles for each girl, so that we could change modestly without the acrobatics required under our dressing gowns in the communal changing-rooms we'd had when we were tiny. Everyone seemed so much more grown up. Once more, I'd arrived in the middle of a school year. I had to learn to fit in, all over again.

We had new uniforms. Sailor hats replaced the old boaters. Tunics, ties, and girdles were shelved in favour of modern pleated skirts and open-necked blouses. The skirts were less hard-wearing and couldn't be sent to the laundry, so we washed them ourselves on Saturday morning, first carefully tacking the pleats to keep them in place, then swishing them up and down in a bathtub filled with soapy hot water that would gradually turn an inky purple. We laid them to dry on our towels over the wall that bisected the Quad. This way, they ended up neat, needing no ironing. The rule was that skirt hems must be no more than four inches off the ground when you were kneeling, but this didn't prevent us from rolling the waistline over two or three times to shorten them.

The Second Vatican Council was in progress, and our nuns were all for modernisation. Over the next couple of years, the liturgy and many of the frills of our religion were transformed. The altar in our Chapel was moved away from the back wall, so the priest could stand behind it, facing us. Mass was no longer in Latin, but in English. Guitars, local drums, and happy-clappy music were introduced, much to our delight. It wasn't long before most of the nuns ditched their drab habits, rosary beads, and wimples for calf-length, lighter dresses, more practical for running around the hockey pitches; and simple cotton veils, which left their hair exposed. We were amazed to discover that nuns actually had hair that could be fair or dark, straight or curly. We no longer referred to the nuns as Mother So-and-So: they were now called Sister.

Fortunately, many of my friends were still there, including Val. We played familiar games. 'Dare, Truth, Kiss, Command or Promise' was still a favourite. In one of the daytime commands, the victim had to sit in a thick column of safari ants: fortunately I was never on the receiving end of that one. One popular dare during rainy season evenings was to go to the bathroom, where the lights were kept on all night, catch one of the hundreds of flying termites that congregated around the light bulbs, remove its wings, and eat it – alive. I remember the creature wriggling in my mouth, the crunch of the squirming exoskeleton between my teeth, the vaguely cheesy flavour. 'Another dare,' Val reminded me recently, 'was to have my ears pierced… you did the honours in the bathroom after lights out with a needle and thread. I still have the holes.' I have no recollection of being brave enough to do this, but Val insists I did, and I'm happy to take the credit. I must have learnt the skill from Silvia.

We now had Swahili in the curriculum, taught by Sister Teresa Joseph – Gorilla. She was small and elderly, a scatty professor-type genius: rumour had it that she had at least three Ph.Ds. When the nuns updated their attire, Gorilla chose to stick with her old-fashioned habit. I loved our Swahili classes, because I found the subject easy. I liked the logic of the spelling, the regular rhythm of the intonation, the patterns of the verb conjugations, the predictable sentence structure.

My father, ever the perfectionist, insisted that we speak what was known as *Kiswahili kisafi* – clean Swahili – rather than the 'kitchen Swahili' used by many *wazungu* – Europeans – which he considered disrespectful. We knew to greet local people older than us with hands together, head bowed, and the word '*Shikamoo*', which literally means 'I touch your leg', to which they responded '*Marahaba*', thanking us for our respect. A glass, to us, was a proper *bilauri*, rather than a corrupted *glassi*.

Gorilla was impressed, and I was proud, because she wasn't easy to please. In our final term of primary school, she put on a play, *Omari Hodari* – Brave Omari. In it, a young girl, Hazina, is depressed and refuses to speak. I was cast as Hazina's mother. I was delighted that Ella of the greasy hair didn't get a part. I had to say '*Mwanangu, Hazina, jaribu kucheka, jaribu kusema*' – 'Hazina, my child, try to laugh, try to speak'. But my entreaties were in vain; Hazina remained downcast and silent… until the dashing Omari danced onto the stage. Hazina's face miraculously lit up. She was cured… and spoke. I wish I could remember what she said.

At Loreto we spoke a unique language containing a hotchpotch of words of various origins. The accent was halfway to that of South African whites. We used several Afrikaans words: tangerines were *naartjes*, and sports shoes were *takkies*. If you felt disappointed, the exclamation was *shame*, and *ag sies* expressed disgust… often heard when one of Matthias' various milk puddings appeared at table. *Voetzek* was an insulting expletive meaning 'Go away'. Marbles were *nyabs*: I have no idea of the etymology of that one.

Our speech was peppered with Swahili words and expressions: whenever you went to visit someone, you would call '*Hodi!*' as you knocked on the door, meaning 'May I come in?' The response was '*Karibu!*' – 'Welcome!' The Paludrine tablets distributed at the beginnings and ends of terms to those of us coming from malarial areas were, to us, malaria *dawa*s. Flying termites, safari ants, and any other insects were *dudu*s.

I will always be grateful to my stars that we were brought up hearing and speaking Italian, English, and Swahili. And our ears were opened to smatterings of so much more: the local languages of the towns where we lived, French in Kigoma, Latin in our prayers and rituals, even a bit of Ancient Greek with our *Kyrie Eleison*s.

Back home with our parents, we would tone down our accents, and eliminate slang and vulgarity, but much of the Swahili stuck, and does to this day. An indispensable word we use is *pole* (**polé** – two syllables), which more or less means *I empathise with your suffering*, used in countless situations ranging from condolences to solidarity with someone walking up a hill or carrying a heavy basket. No English word is as all-encompassing and effective.

While we were in Scotland, Kenya had become independent. Large numbers of white settlers and British passport-holding Asians left the country for the U.K. More African girls started attending the school: there had only been a handful before we went away. As we had done before, we gathered in the Quad for Assembly every Friday – or in the Hall on rainy days – but instead of singing 'God Save our Gracious Queen' and raising the Union Jack decorated with Kenya's red lion, the new Kenyan flag – a black, red, and green tricolour with a red Maasai shield in the middle – was hoisted, and we sang the new national anthem, '*Ee Mungu Nguvu Yetu*'. It was a jerky tune in a minor key, and I didn't find it nearly as moving as our Tanzanian anthem. I remember standing as tall as I could, chest puffed out, turning to grin at Val beside me, as I sang all the verses both in Swahili and English… while Ella, a few places down the line, mimed nonsense.

I was definitely not the newbug here.

Nerone

The year 1966 was an important one: I turned twelve and finished primary school, and after fifteen years in Tanganyika, my father left Government service for the private sector. The new Italian-built oil refinery, TIPER, had been completed, and my father was hired as company doctor for the five hundred employees and their families.

Our lives changed: my parents' fourteenth move in eighteen years of marriage took us to a two-storey (*two-storey*!) house. One wing was my father's waiting room (where Enrico slept) and consulting room. These rooms were air-conditioned. The main part of the house was built on columns, over an open carport, and a verandah, bordered by creepers on the road-facing side, and had an extensive garden – a patch of wasteland as were all our gardens – on the other side. That verandah was our dining room, in the middle of which was the table my parents had found in pieces strewn around the garden.

Upstairs my parents had their air-conditioned bedroom, beside the bathroom. A large living room had been partitioned in two to fashion a bedroom for Silvia and me, cooled by a squeaky fan, which vainly shoved hot air about.

A back door from our bedroom opened outside onto some stairs, which led down to a pokey kitchen and pantry.

My father immediately got down to work in the garden to build our *banda*, a thatched bamboo hut, which was later used for parties and for his regular band practice: he played the mandolin, and a drummer, a guitarist, and a keyboard player, who would later become my brother-in-law, completed the group.

Every morning my father cycled the sixteen kilometres to the refinery, where he saw to patients and their Tanzanian families who lived nearby, and every afternoon he consulted from home for families from the TIPER Village, a new housing complex in Oyster Bay built for the refinery's Italian employees.

While Enrico and Silvia were becoming interested in hanging out with other teenagers and going to parties, I spent a lot of time with Nerone, my Labrador-cross soulmate. We had a deal. We looked after each other.

Our new house was not far from Oyster Bay, and in the mornings we would walk to the beach. Or rather, he would drag me, and I would struggle to hang onto his lead. Over the couple of years he had been with us, he had become increasingly aggressive. On one occasion, he ripped the lead out of my hand, bounded into a neighbour's property, and injured a goat tethered there. We paid twenty shillings for a new goat. Another time, he bit a passer-by, whose injured hand my father sewed up. When he wasn't with me, Nerone was confined to his lead, attached to a long wire in the garden, where he could run up and down. But he was gentle with me, and I felt safe with him.

One morning, while I was walking back home with him from Oyster Bay, thick clouds gathered above us, the air became clammy, and the heavens opened. Waves exploded against the nearby cliffs, and water spilled onto the road. Within minutes we were soaked. My white T-shirt clung to my body, and rivulets dripped from my shorts to my flipflops. Nerone was unperturbed, but I quickened my step and started heading back.

A pale blue Volkswagen Beetle pulled up beside us. The large Indian man at the wheel, hair slicked back, a grin on his face, wound down his window.

'Where are you going?'

'Home. Kinondoni Road.'

'I'll give you a lift.'

I hesitated.

'I'm all wet, I'll mess up your car.'

'No problem. Hop in.'

No. There were rules. Twelve-year-old-girls didn't get into cars with strangers. But it was tempting. The sky hung threateningly low: lightning bolts flashed across the dark sky, followed instantly by deafening thunderclaps. By now the road was a gushing river. I looked homewards, my eyes blurred by rain, then peered into the man's dry car.

'The dog comes in the car too,' I said, surprised by my assertiveness.

'No, he can run behind,' the man replied.

'I'm not allowed to take him off his lead. He stays with me.'

Sighing, the man opened the back door, and Nerone and I got in. I clung onto Nerone's soggy neck and could feel the reassuring vibrations of his growls. The acrid smell of his wet fur mingled with the car's sickly air freshener. The man sped as fast as he could through the puddles to Kinondoni Road, and let us out. I saw him take out a hanky and wipe his sweaty neck as he drove off.

I never told my parents the story. Some things you don't share. I'd broken the rules. It was my secret, and Nerone's.

*

At the beginning of the next school holiday, my mother picked us up from the airport. There was a strange hush, an awkwardness, in the car.

My father was waiting in the carport when we arrived home. We greeted him, and I asked, 'Where's Nerone?'

'We need to talk,' my mother said. 'Let's have some fresh orange.'

And so we all gathered around the dining-room table.

'Don't worry, Nerone is fine,' my father said. 'We had to take a difficult decision. We sent him to a mission in Mbeya.' Mbeya is a town eight hundred kilometres southwest of Dar. 'The priests will look after him.'

'But why?' Jumbled thoughts rushed around in my head. Something here did not add up. Why would they choose a mission that was too far for me to visit? There were plenty of missions nearby.

'He was dangerous. You know that.'

I nodded. I could feel my brow furrowing, and tears filling my eyes.

'He could have killed a child.' My father looked straight at me as he spoke.

And there I shouted, 'He could kill a child in Mbeya too!'

My parents looked at each other. My mother put her arms around me. 'He'll be happy there; he has lots of space to run around in…'

I wanted to grab my glass, still full of orange juice, and smash it on the ground. But there were rules. Twelve-year-olds didn't throw things. So I yelled. 'It's a lie. I'm fed up of being protected. Do you really think I'm too stupid to know what really happened? Stop treating me like a baby.' And I stormed to my room. And sulked for a long time.

On that day I realised that my parents could break rules too: rules of infallibility, wisdom, and honesty. I was not angry at what they had done to Nerone. I understood it was the only solution. But I was angry at their half-baked story. How could I ever trust them again?

It took me many years – perhaps till I was a parent myself – to realise that parents mostly do their best. They do what they think is right. Even if it doesn't always turn out the way they would like.

NAIROBI AND DAR ES SALAAM

1967-1972

The World Beyond

Secondary school was fun, most of the time. We could hold our heads high and lord it over all the primary kids. We became more creative and adventurous. We stretched our dares beyond our primary school limits.

My misdemeanours were mild, but even for the goody-two-shoes among us there was a world beyond school rules, waiting to be discovered.

Making cream cheese became a popular activity. We would save our milk in its bottles for a few days until it curdled, then pour it into clean hankies over a bathtub to let the whey drain off. We'd tie up the hankies and hang them out of the dorm windows for a couple more days. At this point we added the final touches. The bravest amongst us – I only did this once or twice – sneaked out of bounds to the *duka* to buy garlic, onions, and chives. We'd chop them all up and add them to our smelly solidified curds, which we would eat with crackers or bread filched from the dining room. The effort we put into it made our cheese all the more delicious.

One day a few of us decided to make peanut brittle for a midnight feast. This required a fair amount of *duka* shopping: sugar, butter, and peanuts. The sugar had to be melted, and organising this step required pluck. The chemistry labs, which were upstairs, were kept locked. After dark, a friend and I climbed out of the window of the dorm adjoining the lab, crept along a ledge, in through the lab window, grabbed a couple of Bunsen burners, and slunk back. After lights out we set to work, chopping nuts and melting butter and sugar in pots improvised from tins.

Tap, tap, tap… footsteps… the Head Girl!

'What do you think you're doing?'

Six of us, huddled around the Bunsen burners between two beds, froze. Fortunately, the Head Girl's sister was one of our gang, so the incident went unreported. I can't imagine what the punishment would have been for this serious and dangerous offence. I will never forget the heart-stopping tingle that came with these escapades.

Once, simply for being caught talking after lights out, we were all made to stand in the chilly Quad in our nighties for what seemed like hours. My friend Anna remembers that the nun who punished us said, 'Those who shield the guilty will be struck by lightning'. The next day, we were made to write letters home.

Dear Mummy and Daddy,

I don't deserve the golden place I have in this school…

Sister Germaine, who was our headmistress at the time, had used this as a scare tactic, and the letters were not sent.

In class, I enjoyed doing well, but didn't put myself out too much. I suppose I was a typical adolescent with a bit of an attitude. I learnt that the way to star effortlessly was to give up subjects that required too much study and stick with the ones that came easily. One advantage of being at boarding school was that it wasn't easy for our parents to keep track of what we were up to: they didn't attend teachers' meetings or have the opportunity to talk to us about homework or assignments. I played the nuns and my parents off each other: 'Oh mamma, the Latin teacher is sooo boooring!' 'Yes, Sister, my parents say I can give up chemistry.' 'Mamma, there's so much homework; I don't have time to practise the piano...' Sheer laziness, because I wasn't actually a disaster at all those subjects. 'You were good at Latin,' my friend Alison remembers. 'During exams you would pass your answers around the class, and we would adjust a bit here and there...'

I must have inherited this helpful trait from my parents, both of whom told stories of doing their classmates' homework for them and sending answers around on notes in class.

By the time I reached 'O' levels, Latin, History, Physics, Chemistry, and Music had all fallen by the wayside. And since our years were streamed, I didn't do Drama, Needlework or Domestic Science either.

In my defence, I missed chunks of school through no fault of my own, which didn't help my motivation. When I was fifteen, I became ill with a throat infection a week before half-term and was put in isolation in the infirmary: no visitors allowed. I was feverish and miserable. None of the dragon nursing sister's lotions and potions worked, and in about ten days my weight dropped from forty-five to forty kilos. My best friend Christina sneaked in to see me one day.

'Call Germaine,' I croaked.

Sister Germaine was aghast when she saw me. She sat on my iron-framed bed and gently put her hand on my forehead.

'You're going home,' she said. An air ticket was bought, I was whisked off to the airport, and was soon tucked up in my bed in Dar, with my father taking swabs, getting lab tests, and administering the right antibiotics. Within days I was better, but my mother decided to keep me home for the rest of term.

The following year, Silvia got married six weeks before the end of term. I went home for the celebrations, and once again, my parents kept me there.

My marks suffered from my absences. I kept on with Biology because we were required to take one science subject. I wasn't particularly good at it, but enjoyed the practical side, when we dissected ant lions and cow's eyes. Once we were all taken outside to pick a moonflower to dissect. The entire class ended up in the infirmary with swollen eyes and dilated pupils... how did the teacher not know that moonflowers are toxic?

Sports and swimming were not my forte, but I enjoyed them and tried my best. Once I flukily managed to wangle my way onto a hockey team. I played right inner, a safe position where you didn't have to bully off, or take free hits, but could just hide amongst the others. Our teacher was Hikey – Sister Hyacinth – a wonderfully energetic woman who wore a leaf tucked between her glasses and the bridge of her nose to protect it from the sun, and went on to live till she was 102.

The three Italian boarders in my class, Anna, Marta, and I, attended private Italian classes given by Mrs. Moretti, the mother of a day girl at our school. This was the highlight of our week: it involved leaving the school grounds, taking a public bus, and getting ourselves to Mrs. Moretti's home. She was a lovely woman, impeccably elegant. Her only concession to imperfection was a few hairpins that stuck out of her neatly pleated blonde bun. The temptation to reach out and push them in was overpowering.

Marta remembers Mrs. Moretti's explanation of *il futuro nel passato* – the future in the past. 'She would fling an arm forward (into the future) like swimming crawl, jabbing with her index finger, and then proceed to use her thumb to point backwards over her head into the past.'

Anna recalls 'her long blood-red nails, and above all that she offered us tea and biscuits. We were always hungry. It was an occasion to get out. Sometimes we stopped on the way back to school for an ice-cream.' Italian classes were a genuine treat.

My parents expected good results from us, but they didn't have high ambitions for Silvia and me. Enrico was to go to Italy and study civil engineering. Silvia and I could go for higher studies if we wanted to, but I will never forget my mother telling me that, once I was married (this step was taken for granted), since I was good at languages, I could get a *lavoretto* – a little job that would keep me amused.

French was by far the easiest subject for me. In my early secondary years, we had a teacher, Polish I think, with no neck and a long name beginning with Z and ending with *–ski*. She would invariably waddle into the classroom and say, 'Papers and pencils ready: *Dictée.*' She would proceed to dictate a paragraph from a book, then say, 'Exchange books with your neighbour. Except you, Paola. Come and write the dictation on the board.' I wasn't bothered; it passed the time pleasantly enough. No one seemed to mind my being teacher's pet… it saved them a lot of hassle.

Mrs. Z. didn't last long and, leading up to our Cambridge 'O' levels, we had a series of unmemorable teachers. The result was that sixteen pupils out of the twenty-two who sat the French exam failed miserably.

For a few weeks we had a half-decent French teacher who taught us Jacques Prévert's poem, *Page d'Ecriture*. By that stage many of the class were beyond caring, but I was captivated:

Deux et deux quatre
Quatre et quatre huit
Huit et huit font seize
Répétez! dit le maître

Or, in English:

Two and two four
Four and four eight
Eight and eight make sixteen
Once again! says the master

I recognised the scenario: it was Mrs. Z all over…

But then, in the poem, a bird comes down through the window and plays with the child, who says:

Save me
Play with me
Bird…

And despite the teacher's entreaties:

… the window panes return to sand
The ink returns to water
The desks return to trees
The chalk returns to the mines
The feather quill returns to the bird

… and I could float out through the window to a world where classroom walls fade away, far beyond school uniforms, far beyond the boundaries of our school, far beyond buying garlic at the *duka*, far beyond even Mrs. Moretti's living room, to another world, where children could be free to dream in whatever language they chose amongst sand and water and trees and birds.

Teenagers and Tek-Teks

Let's go surfin' now
Everybody's learning how
Come on and safari with me

Music blared from a transistor radio as we sped along in our friend Carlo's jeep, singing along with the Beach Boys at the tops of our voices, tapping the sides of the car, the wind in our hair. The older teenagers tolerated us younger siblings, and life was fun. Our holidays were one big party. For several weeks, nine hundred kilometres separated us, body and mind, from school, homework, nuns, and priests.

We gathered in groups at the beach, body surfed (no one had real surfboards), and got sunburnt. We would compete to see who could peel the largest piece of flaky skin off each other's backs.

Enrico took up spearfishing, but my mother didn't like him going alone, so if he didn't have a companion, Silvia or I would go with him. I remember baking under the blistering sun far out to sea at Oyster Bay as I sat rocking in the waves in an inflated inner tube, which was attached by a rope to Enrico's waist. I cannot begin to imagine what I would have done in an emergency. He would surface every now and then with catches of rock-cod, parrotfish, stingrays, moray eels, and even lobsters. (He told me recently that the lobsters were occasionally filched from fishermen's lobster traps.) My mother would delight in making us exquisite *fritti misti* and *bouillabaisse* with his hauls.

Enrico had a Lambretta – he would have liked a motorbike but my mother didn't approve.

'Let's go for a spin!' he'd say, and I'd leap onto the back, helmetless like he was, and cling on tight to him as he swooped and skidded around dusty bends yelling, 'Lean the corners! You have to lean the corners or we'll fall!'

In the evenings we kids sometimes went to the drive-in, our car packed, hiding a couple of extra people in the boot to get them in free. On the way we'd sing, in our best South African accents, Jeremy Taylor's recent hit, 'Ag Pleez Deddy':

Ag pleez Deddy won't you take us to the drive-in
All six, seven of us, eight, nine, ten
We wanna see a flick about
Tarzan an' the Ape-men
An' when the show is over you can bring us back again

There was a seating area at the back where you could buy popcorn. At weekends Bollywood movies would play.

'Hindi movie!' the baffled-looking people in the next car would call to us.

'We know! We know!' And we'd sing along in Hindi to *Jab Jab Bahar Aaye*, with no clue what the lyrics meant, and giggle at the suggestive peeping-from-behind-flowery-bushes glances on the screen.

When I was around fifteen my parents began allowing me to go to teenage parties, dressed in outfits made by Silvia from fabrics haggled over in the Indian quarter. She had a real talent, and I was happy to assist as she fashioned collars and pockets and buttonholes and sewed on sequins and braided borders. The parties were held in clubs or private homes, and the flurry of nerves and hormones almost outweighed my feelings of ignorance, inadequacy, and humiliation as I observed the heady haze from the sidelines with my friends, simultaneously praying that someone would ask me to dance, and that they wouldn't. When I was sixteen both Enrico and Silvia got married… and I was left on my own, without their protection.

An Indian photographer called Mr. Mistri attended these events, taking his camera from dance floor to bar to dark corners of the garden, and a couple of days later, we would traipse off to his shop, flip through his album marked 'ADUALTS ARE NOT ALOWED TO LOOK IN THIS BOOK', and order prints.

As the years drifted by, home, school, home, school, home, different clans formed. A few people started gathering under the palm trees at the far end of Oyster Bay, smoking.

'Why are they always dressed in black?' my mother would ask. 'Why do they face the road, with their backs to the ocean?' I don't think they really cared what they wore or what view they had. The earthy, herbal scent that enveloped them was definitely not tobacco. Marijuana grew wild in some of our friends' gardens, and could be bought cheaply at the frenzied Kariakoo Market, where amongst honking horns and hawkers calling '*Papai*! Pawpaw! *Embe*! Mango!' whispers of 'Change money? Dollar? Good price!' alternated with '*Banghi, Banghi*!'

Our taste in music moved on from the Beach Boys to the Mamas and Papas to The Doors and Jefferson Airplane. I never joined the crowd at the far end of Oyster Bay. Fortunately, I was too much of a wimp. I say fortunately, because many of the black-clad gang moved on from hash to harder stuff, and paid for it in later life. The crescendo in the final lines of Jefferson Airplane's 'White Rabbit' fed my head and safely lifted me as high as I wanted to be.

When logic and proportion
Have fallen sloppy dead
And the White Knight is talking backwards
And the Red Queen's off with her head
Remember what the dormouse said
Feed your head
Feed your head

*

Weekends were family time. For a long time, my mother and I continued to go to Mass at St. Peter's Church as the others dropped out one by one. One day I asked her, 'Mamma, why do you go to Mass?' 'For you,' she answered. And I'd been going for her. So we stopped, which meant the whole family could spend longer at the beach. I say 'the beach' but there was a vast range of possible venues, and we would choose depending on the day's planned activity, which in turn depended on the tide. We became tide experts and studied the tables in our local paper.

Twice a month, at neap tide, from one hour before high tide to one hour after, it was *tek-tek*-catching time. What we called *tek-teks* were rainbow-coloured bivalves belonging to a species of mini-clam called *donax*. They lived on the shoreline of beaches that were far from any reefs. We would cross the harbour on the ferry and drive to Mjimwema, a village where we could rent a beach hut for the day for five shillings. It was quiet: no parasols, no deckchairs, no ice-cream sellers, no one hawking crafts, just balmy air, palm trees, and a few fishermen in the hazy distance bringing in their catch. And us, in an immensity of bleached sand and sparkling sea. My father didn't like the sun and would spend the day reading and sleeping in the hut, while the rest of us sat on the lace-edged tideline, the warm waves lapping around our thighs, our hands scratching under the sand till we touched something hard… a *tek-

tek burrowing away. We had competitions to see how many *tek-teks* we would find in ten minutes, or who would be the first to fill a plastic cup, which we would then empty into a bucket of sea water.

Back home, the *tek-tek*s would be left for a few hours in the water to spit out all their sand, then my mother would fry them up with some garlic and tomatoes and make a delicious sauce to go with her home-made pasta. *Spaghetti alle vongole.* Yum.

Champagne Socialism

The fold-up table was like a large, heavy suitcase, and incorporated two benches that emerged from its rusty workings of hinges and slats when you opened it. Its sandpapery top and seats were a pale aquamarine, shimmery and uneven in colour, like tide pools. My father heaved it into the boot of the burnt-orange Ford Cortina. Enrico followed, his arms laden with his harpoon gun, and mismatching flippers and goggles. Silvia dragged a huge towel-filled *kikapu* – basket – along the ground. I helped my mother fill up a cool box with Cokes. And a couple of limes. And our last precious bottle of olive oil. And bags of ice cubes. And a small hammer. And finally, a bottle of champagne.

Our adolescent and teenage years coincided with President Julius Nyerere's implementation of his idealistic *Ujamaa* policy, modelled on Chinese socialism. *Ujamaa* can be roughly translated as 'togetherness'. He installed a one-party system, and by the early seventies, millions of people had been moved from their homes to new *Ujamaa* villages, which were designed to foster self-reliance. Although the country benefited in many ways – infant mortality was reduced, school enrolment soared – *Ujamaa* ultimately failed, for many reasons ranging from the 1970s oil crisis to drought, corruption and lack of foreign investment.

We, the privileged Europeans, felt the effects in Dar. Many day-to-day commodities were often in short supply, and people like us, fortunate enough to be able to travel, would come home with our suitcases filled with light bulbs bought in Kenya at the end of one term, and toilet paper at the end of the next. Some of the contents of our suitcases were useful as 'gifts' to customs officials to speed up luggage checks on entering the country.

My mother had found a job at the French Embassy, next door to our house, and benefited from diplomatic privileges (or rather, I imagine that as a local employee she cashed in on someone else's diplomatic allowance). So, whilst it might be difficult to find sugar or coffee in the shops, she was able to order duty-free goods. Which is why we had champagne.

We lugged the cool box through the verandah to the carport, holding it underneath, as the plastic handle was broken. We piled into the car, my father and Enrico in shorts and T-shirts, and we three girls wearing brightly-coloured *kanga*s over our bathing suits. Every *kanga* typically had a proverb printed on it. Mine said '*Usiposiba ufa, utajenga ukuta*', which means 'If you don't fix the hole, you'll need to build a wall'. The brakes squeaked and the doors rattled as we juddered north through two rows of tall, orange-blossomed flamboyant trees on the bumpy track to Msasani Bay, and I wondered if my proverb applied to cars and picnic tables and cool boxes.

We had consulted the tide tables in the *Daily News*, and today, low spring tide fell at around midday. We reached Msasani Bay and parked under the fringing palm trees. A dozen or so fishermen crowded around the car, vying for custom. A sweet blend of sweat, salt, seaweed, and fish filled the air.

'Bongoyo? Mbudya?'

Bongoyo and Mbudya were small uninhabited islands a couple of kilometres off the coast, popular with day-trippers, who generally sailed or hired a speedboat to take them there at weekends from the Dar Yacht Club, or the new elegant government-built hotels along Kunduchi Beach to the north of the city. Each of these islands had sparkling white beaches, and fishermen would bring in their fish, cook them on open fires, and serve them to sunburnt visitors.

We had discovered that the fishermen at Msasani Beach, halfway between the Yacht Club and the fancy hotels, were happy to take us across in their *ngalawas* – traditional double-outrigger canoes made from hollowed-out mango trees. It was a longer trip, but it was cheaper, and so much more fun.

'*Salaam alaikum*,' my mother said.

'Bongoyo? Mbudya? Good wind! New sail! Mbudya? Bongoyo?'

But we had other plans. 'Pangavini.'

Pangavini was a tiny, mushroom-shaped coral island between Mbudya and Bongoyo, which could only be reached at low tide when its beach was exposed. No one went there, apart from a few fishermen and us. It couldn't be accessed at high tide, when breakers crashed against its cliffs. After some lively haggling, my mother reached a deal with a fisherman called Musa.

At high tide the *ngalawa*s were dragged up onto the beach, but at low tide they were anchored a long way out, and we traipsed with our bags and equipment across a couple of hundred yards of intertidal mudflats, our rubber flipflops slurping in the wet sand, we kids stopping occasionally, to dump our cargo, and pick up a brittle star and watch it crawl over our hands.

We were puffed when we reached the *ngalawa*. We scrambled in, and Musa pushed the boat out into the water. He climbed in and handed us each a rusty, holey tin to help bail out the water that came through the cracks in the hull. It was calm, luckily, and a gentle breeze cooled our sweaty skins. Every time Musa tacked, Enrico and Silvia, who were sitting near the boom, had to climb over it, which made the boat wobble, and my mother would squeal '*Oddio!*'

When we reached Pangavini, we had to cross a hundred yards or so of coral reef and tide pools to reach the now exposed sandy cove. We trod carefully around sea urchins, their eye-like googly anuses staring up at us. Pink sea anemones waved their fronds in the transparent water. Bobbly seaweed floated to the surface. Silvia burst a bobble and rubbed the gooey liquid on her skin. 'It's as good as aloe,' she said.

At last we were settled on the beach. Musa waved good-bye.

'*Tutaonana*,' he said. See you later. And off he sailed. And we simply trusted that he would return. A particularly low low tide, like today's, meant an exceptionally high high tide, and when the water came in, Pangavini would become a waterlocked outcrop with no beach.

My mother took out the olive oil and we slathered our skins with it: the theory was that this would moisturise it and give us a healthy tan. My father, as usual, spent the day dozing or reading in the shade – at Pangavini this meant in a cave, as there were no palm trees. Enrico walked backwards in his flippers lugging his fishing equipment across the coral to the water. Silvia and I followed my mother to the coral heads fringing the island, carrying the hammer, the bottle of champagne, the chopped limes, and some plastic cups.

And there they were, in their thousands: big, juicy oysters embedded in the coral, looking as though they had been there since prehistory. In turn, we took the hammer, tapped a tightly clamped zigzag joint, prised the oyster open, squeezed on a drop of lime, and scooped out the slimy flesh with our fingers, swallowing each oyster whole. Oh, so sweet, so tangy, so salty! And between each oyster, we took a sip of champagne.

'Go and wet your hair now,' my mother said. This was another family theory: wetting your hair prevented you from getting sunstroke.

Soon Enrico was back with his haul: today he'd caught two small lobsters, a stingray, and three rock cod. This would be our feast tonight.

The water began to rise, slipping across the tide pools, spreading a smooth, buttery layer over the sea urchin spikes and rocky protuberances. We gazed shorewards, sipping champagne from plastic cups – apart from my father who was a teetotaller for his entire long life – and a spot moving towards us from the beach came into focus, gradually transforming into Musa with his *ngalawa*.

And so we headed back to the shore and the car, no lighter than when we'd left in the morning, with sand in our hair and our swimsuits and our *kikapu*, Enrico's catch having replaced the champagne, tired, burnt, happy, and most of us slightly tipsy. Supermarket shelves might be empty, but for us teenagers, life was good.

What Lies Beneath

Helvola Argella was my favourite. The star cowrie. Sparkling, speckled, it evoked a moonless African night. Its base was a startling violet.

As teenagers we were passionate about cowries. We collected, cleaned, classified and traded them around the world, with fellow-subscribers to a magazine called *Hawaiian Shell News*. We would send our finds off to exotic places such as Guam and Malaysia. Weeks later we would open our P.O. Box at the dusty Central Post Office and squeal with delight at finding a padded envelope containing a sub-species we'd never seen before.

Cowries have been prized for their patterns, colour, and shape for centuries. Hundreds of years ago, the common money cowrie was used as currency in parts of Asia and Africa. By the eighteenth century, tons of cowries were being exchanged for boatloads of slaves.

Today, rare cowries are cherished by collectors. In the fashion industry, they decorate belts, sandals, and jewellery. There are over two hundred cowrie species living in tropical and sub-tropical waters, varying from under ten millimetres to almost twenty centimetres in length, and from near snow white to jet black.

Cowrie shells have little commercial value unless they are collected alive. Without their mollusc clinging to a rock, the waves toss them about and they crack, and lose their shine.

With a group of half a dozen friends, we would explore reefs that were only exposed at low spring tides. These fell every two weeks for a couple of days, between 11 a.m. and 1 p.m.

We slapped on hats, slipped on T-shirts over our swimsuits, and slopped olive oil onto our skins. We wore our scruffiest trainers and tied specially fashioned plastic jars around our waists with string. We carried iron bars, which were forged with a hook on the end, to turn stones.

Over forty species of cowrie have been identified in the Dar area. At first we used a basic printed guide called *Collecting Cowries in Dar es Salaam*, which contained faded black and white photos and brief descriptions, but soon our combined knowledge and experience surpassed the authors'. We learnt all the cowrie names in Latin and English, and knew exactly where we were likely to find each species. Few could be seen crawling on the open reef. Only the common Money and Gold-ringed Cowries, and the misnamed black and white spotted Tiger Cowrie didn't mind being exposed to the sun.

We found most cowries clinging upside down under large rocks, along with brittle stars, anemones, squids, sea cucumbers and eels. But some were particular about their habitat: the black-based oval yellow banded Mole Cowrie chose flat slabs, while the dark Arabian Cowrie hid in the rocky recesses of massive boulders, along with the web-patterned Harlequin, and occasionally, the rarer, purple-based Mauritania. The small Snake's Head tucked itself into tiny holes on these same boulders, where it was well camouflaged. The black Onyx preferred muddy surroundings, as did the yellow and green spotted Lamarck, and these clung to rotting poles in murkier waters where the fishermen attached their nets.

Occasionally we braved the stink of the sewage pipe, which

stretched out to sea on the mudflats opposite the Ocean Road Hospital. Years before, a ship had lost a cargo of tiles there, and under the slimy pieces of ceramic, you could find the rare Stolida Cowrie, grey with a brown rectangle on its back.

Often the cowries were covered by their mantle, a protective film. The Sieve Cowrie's mantle was a tangerine orange.

We learnt that some, like the coveted Argus, with its mini hula-hoop ring patterns, lived below the intertidal mark, deep in tightly packed red organ coral. To hunt for these, we would go by boat to an underwater reef called Fungu Mkadya, don flippers and snorkels, and – I squirm when I think of this – gently pull apart the branches of coral. In five years, I only ever found one Argus.

We did not question what we were doing. We felt that it was legitimate. We had our Code of Conduct, based on the one upheld by *Hawaiian Shell News*:

- Leave live coral heads alone. Look in the rubble, under the slabs, in the sand and amongst loose chunks.
- Put rocks and coral back in place, where you found them, even in deep water.
- Be alert for eggs and protect them. Never take a mollusc that is guarding them.
- Collect only what you need.
- Never take an immature specimen.

Back home, tired, our skin salt-and-sun-tight, our containers filled with the day's catch, the cleaning operation would start. Again I shudder at the memory. *Collecting Cowries in Dar es Salaam* nonchalantly informed us that the shells were to be left rotting in kerosene for three days, after which the animal could be squirted out with a strong jet from a hosepipe. When they were clean, we dried and labelled them, and stored them in dark drawers so they wouldn't fade.

It was an unusual hobby. Our parents were pleased that we were indulging in a wholesome activity that kept us from the pale, hash-puffing crowd who spent their days lolling under the palm trees in a foggy stupor.

Thirty years later, I returned to Dar as an accompanying spouse. Here was an opportunity to expiate my crimes. I went to the National Museum to see if I could do something in the field of environmental protection, or community education.

'Oh yes, we are trying to classify our shells,' a museum official told me. He took me to a room where dusty shelves were weighed down with hundreds of plastic bags filled with a jumble of dirty, stinking shells.

'These aren't very good,' he said. 'You seem to know what you're talking about. Why don't you collect more and bring them to us?' I went home feeling nauseous, and never returned to the museum.

Exploring my old haunts, I found that in many places, our beautiful coral reefs had become vast stretches of rubble, the result of dynamite fishing. Fishermen had discovered that with a quick blast, entire shoals of fish would die and float to the surface. In one of the poorest countries in the world, it is no wonder that the survival of coral reefs and pretty shells was hardly a priority.

Luckily, other areas were unspoilt. My passion for cowrie shells was as alive as ever, but it had become deeper, more discerning. I still scrutinised the tide tables and visited the reefs at low tide.

For four years, I worked on a new shell collection. I took photos of live cowries in their natural environment: encouraging evidence that at least some of these treasures were still alive and reproducing, despite the pressures from fishermen and souvenir shoppers.

And I wrote these lines:

What Lies Beneath

Helvola Argella's Milky Way shell
shields her fragile body, as she scours
coral for a mate;

Sun-withered Baraka raises
hope-filled candle high:
boom! Fish float, broken in froth;

Helvola Argella, cracked and dull,
mate-date hopes shattered
crawls across war-torn rubble.

Baraka's family will eat tonight.

I wonder how many people realise that if they buy a shiny shell, that shell has most probably been taken alive from its natural habitat.

'A' Level Years

Heavy breathing. Groans and sighs.

Jane Birkin whispers, '*Je t'aime…*'

Serge Gainsbourg responds, '*Moi non plus…*'

We turn up the volume of the record player. This is the smoothest, most sensual song we have ever heard. The organ soars in the background, and our heartbeats quicken.

Someone has managed to get hold of the 45 r.p.m. hit; it will soon be banned.

'*Oh, mon amour, tu es la vague, moi l'île nue*', we pant, giggling.

'You are the wave; I, the naked island,' I translate.

Footsteps. The door opens. Oh, no, Sister Caitriona!

'What's this you're listening to, girls?'

Someone snatches at the record player arm, scratching the record.

'Um… not sure… it's in French… language practice…'

*

Sister Caitriona was our headmistress for our 'A' level years. We adored her. Young, bubbly, with a great sense of humour, she was warm-hearted and always stood up for anyone who was victimised or disadvantaged. Her inclusiveness and avant-garde ideas marked us all for life.

But we gave her a hard time. Once I bumped into her in a corridor. She'd found a suspect item in someone's drawer.

'Is this what I think it is, Paola dear?' she asked me, opening her fist to reveal a rolled-up, transparent teat-like object. I was seventeen and had no idea what she might think it was, nor what it was.

Demographics at Loreto changed considerably in our last years.

The schools in Kenya had recently changed the 'O' level exams from 'Cambridge School Certificate' to 'Kenya School Certificate'. Although the exam papers were still set and marked in Cambridge, many parents felt that they were less prestigious, and moved their children to boarding schools in England. Val, my first friend, left, though we remained in touch.

In 1971, Idi Amin staged a bloody coup in Uganda. Many people fled the country, and our school took in several daughters of officials from the overthrown government. I remember them arriving in the classroom, looking shaken, several weeks after the start of term. 'Don't ask them about what happened,' the nuns told us. 'Just listen if they want to talk to you.'

Few girls stayed on at school for 'A' levels. In those days 'O' levels were considered good enough for girls, and many left for secretarial colleges in Nairobi, or finishing schools in Switzerland, depending on their economic circumstances.

A wonderful, flamboyant woman, Mrs. Dunn, glided into the classroom to teach us English Literature. She wore long cotton skirts that looked as though they had been fashioned from old curtains, and her straw-like hair was always dishevelled. Her magenta spectacle frames pointed upwards at the sides, giving her a startled look. She ranted and raved, laughed and cried, and initially delighted in ripping up our work in front of us. 'Think, girls!' she'd screech. 'Think! No platitudes, please!' It was no surprise when we later learnt that she wasn't an English teacher at all, but a drama teacher. We soon got used to her and ended up loving her. She spent two years instilling in us the techniques which would enable us to give impressive answers to whatever question was on the exam paper, and the entire class of nine girls came out with As and Bs.

During our first year of 'A' levels, Sister Caitriona brought in a handsome, balding priest with dark, deep-set eyes to talk to us about comparative religions. I don't recall his name: let's call him Father O'Donnell. He wasn't a familiar face from St. Mary's next door; he was a scary university lecturer.

I was beginning to question the ideas about religion that had taken shape in my head over the years. It no longer felt right that the world population should be divided into three categories: Catholics (the goodies); non-Catholics (the baddies) who might be Protestants, Muslims or Hindus; and Pagans (who, through no fault of their own, hadn't heard about Jesus and might, if they were lucky, end up in Limbo with unbaptised babies).

We looked forward to Father O'Donnell's classes: he lifted our minds to places they had never before reached. Every week he told us about a different religion. He was offhand and impersonal, plying us with engaging facts and figures. We learnt that Zoroastrians believed in one God and followed the principles of good thoughts, words and deeds. Bahá'ís strove for world peace and equality. Jains were vegetarians and believed in non-violence. What was wrong with that, I wondered. It occurred to me that at schools in faraway Asian countries, pupils learnt about their religion, and not about ours: perhaps we Catholics weren't the centre of the world after all.

One day, Father O'Donnell swooped into the classroom, stood in front of us and asked, 'Do you think you are important? Hands up if you think you are important.'

My hand shot up. Of course I was important. God had made me for a purpose: to know Him, to love Him and to serve Him (although I was beginning to wonder what those words actually meant… and hadn't He made all the Zoroastrians and Jains and Bahá'ís too?).

'You?' Father O'Donnell pointed at me. 'You think you are important?' I felt a warm blush rising to my cheeks. He scanned the upturned faces of my classmates. 'This girl thinks she's important.' He didn't even know my name. 'Girls, think for a moment. Imagine you were in this classroom, and the young lady who just put up her hand wasn't here. She'd never been here. She wasn't a pupil at this school. You'd never met her. She was less than a speck of dust. In fact, she'd never been born. Would you know? Would you care?'

Stunned silence in the classroom. I was crushed. And I never forgot those words.

That same year, Sister Caitriona invited a touring American Christian folk group to sing for us. There were five of them, all blond, all long-haired, all smiley, and, to us, all gorgeous, especially the boys. And, strangely, they were all Protestants.

'It's all the same,' Sister Caitriona said. 'They are good people.'

Again, our eyes were opened to novelty, to a new sincerity and warmth; we were swept away, and wept tears of emotion as we held hands in the Hall, singing 'Kumbaya', 'Peace Like a River', and 'He's Got the Whole World in His Hands'.

'It's all there, in the Bible,' they told us. 'The answer to every question you ever had.'

After Nairobi, they were going to sing in Dar. I wrote to my parents. 'Go and listen to them. They have all the answers.'

My parents went. My father was not impressed, and told me so. My mother was marginally more polite, but not convinced.

The group had said we could write to them with any doubts or queries: they would send us the Bible reference that would clarify everything. I clung on to their words, and wrote to them, asking them how they felt about people of other faiths, and what the Bible had to say on the subject. They never answered.

The struggle in my mind between hope and doubt continued. Finally, doubt won, and I gave up trying. Perhaps it was Father O'Donnell who led me there. Perhaps it was my disappointment in the Holy Huddle group. Perhaps it was Mrs. Dunn's 'Think, girls!' Perhaps Sister Caitriona's innovative ideas encouraged me to question 'my' truth; I will always be grateful to her for this. Perhaps it was all of these. Or perhaps it was simply time.

In my final term at school, I went to Confession. Father Campbell, a gentle, softly spoken priest, sat in the dark confessional.

'Father, I'm coming to tell you that this is my last Confession. I just can't do it any more. I've tried to find the answers: they're not there. I don't understand why I need to come here and tell you my sins, whatever those may be. Why can't I just acknowledge my weaknesses to myself? I can understand values, and principles, and morals, but I can't take the trimmings. I can't take the bits that don't add up.'

'I will pray for you, my child.'

'I can even take prayer,' I said. 'Prayer makes sense.'

Pauline and the Pool

Dozens of Loreto alumnae contacted me when they read about Sister Pauline in my blog, telling me how deeply she had touched their lives: this chapter is for them, and for her.

When I think back to my eleven years of Loreto education, I am filled with appreciation for everything the nuns did for us: they sacrificed their freedom and families to work far from their homes, looking after us. For nine months of the year, they replaced our parents, influencing our values, our outlooks, and our social development.

Of all the nuns I came in contact with, one became a good friend: Sister Pauline. Looking back fifty years to my young self, I ask myself what drew us together, and what keeps us close even when we are continents apart.

In 1970, when I was sixteen and disgruntled, Sister Pauline arrived at Loreto. She was different from the other nuns. She wasn't Irish: she had been brought up in Uganda, a middlish sibling of an English ophthalmologist's ten children. She had an East African accent, like ours. None of the 'Ah sure, pet' Dublinese that her fellow nuns managed to cling on to even after decades on the equator. It was rumoured that Sister Pauline was a psychology graduate.

Until her arrival, nuns were a blurry group, not individuals who may have had parents or siblings or interests. Randomly to us, one taught Geography and another Maths or Scripture. They hollered and stomped. But Sister Pauline didn't holler or stomp. She was one of the first to discard her habit, wimple and clunky beads in favour of a light dress and a veil pushed back to expose a few strands of hair. She was timeless. And minuscule. She spoke in a whisper. Her deep-set eyes seemed to pierce through to the secrets of our adolescent souls. Her quietness made her the most terrifying nun I had met in all my years at boarding school. During our time, Sister Pauline didn't have a nickname; she was simply herself. After I had left school, she became known as Power.

For two years, she was headmistress. I lay low, dreading what might befall me if I got on her wrong side. During her tenure, some of my classmates were expelled for smoking, an activity that never remotely attracted me.

*

After I left school, as I constructed my adult life far from East Africa, I didn't keep in touch with Sister Pauline and the other nuns, apart from one brief visit when I was in Nairobi for a conference twenty years later.

Serendipity reunited us when, in 2000, my husband Willie was posted to Dar. I heard that Sister Pauline, along with a couple of Kenyan nuns, was at a new Loreto Convent that had opened in the poor suburb of Nyakato near Mwanza, on Lake Victoria. I got in touch, and there began the next phase of our relationship. We became good friends.

She stayed with us whenever she was in the capital trying to obtain work permits for her Kenyan teachers.

'Paola dear, you have a pool!' she said, the first time she visited. 'I didn't bring my bathing costume!' I handed her the smallest one

I had. She visibly glowed, and a few moments later had changed into it. Splash! A neat racing dive and twenty lengths of crawl later she emerged. A nun swimming! And not such a young one at that!

On that visit we wandered around Kariakoo market and bought two hundred bras for her pupils. 'I need to get them a useful gift,' she said.

I visited her at Nyakato, and was delighted to see the girls neatly dressed in white blouses and burgundy skirts, just as tidy as we had been at school decades earlier, complete with white ankle socks and polished black shoes, singing the school hymn and the Tanzanian national anthem at Assembly. But Loreto Nyakato was a far cry from Loreto Msongari.

'They have two uniforms each,' Sister Pauline told me, 'and little else in the way of clothes. So many of them are AIDs orphans, you know, but the uniform gives them pride.'

She had introduced a 'foundation year', in which the girls studied English intensively before entering secondary school. This helped with the transition from Swahili to English as the language of education, and proved to be a great success.

Her dream was to build a swimming pool at Nyakato. 'A pool! What a crazy idea!' the sceptics, including my mother, said. 'What do you need a pool for in a poor area?' But, eventually, long after I had left Tanzania, build a pool she did.

We remained in touch by email. She stayed when she came to Brussels some years later and we motored around Germany and the Netherlands together on a fund-raising mission.

A few years ago, when we were living in Ghana, I had an urge see her again, and wrote to her.

Dear Sister Pauline,
I would so like to visit you at Nyakato.
    Lots of love from Paola

I received an immediate reply:

Paola, how wonderful. Please do come and stay and let us have some time together... You will be so welcome, and how lovely to have that to look forward to. You will stay with us and we shall meet you and take care of you. Bring your swimming costume!
Love,
(Sr) Pauline Boase

I loved the way she always put 'Sr' in brackets, as though it didn't count.

Sadly, that trip didn't work out. But a short while later she visited me again in Brussels. I met her at the Eurostar. A slip of a woman, dressed in a blue skirt and white blouse, as unfading as ever, pulling a tiny scarlet case behind her. For two days we played Scrabble, watched the World Cup, and chatted and chatted and chatted. On her request, we went to the Grand-Place and ate *frites* with mayonnaise.

At the end of her trip, we had a hairy ride to the airport. I managed to get us on the wrong train, and we landed up in the middle of Flanders, standing on a deserted platform with her feather-light case. We arrived at the airport with little time to spare, and as we milled through armed soldiers with holiday-spirited throngs, for the first time in my life I saw a cloud flit across her face. 'Paola dear, which piece of paper do I need to show?' I hugged her, scanned her boarding pass, and shoved her through to the security checks at the last minute.

I dashed to her airline desk. 'I have a friend who may miss her flight,' I explained. 'I think she may be anxious...' The official promised to have someone look out for her and got back to me a few minutes later.

'Oh, she made it fine. She was right at the front of the queue. Smiling and happy, with her red case. Refused all help. Turned down our offer of a wheelchair.'

Sister Pauline has always been there for me, with exactly the right words. When my mother died, she wrote:

I shall keep her in my prayers, though I am sure her prayers will be much more useful to us.

And three years later:

Thank you, dear Paola, for letting me know of your father's death. He did not linger on too long after your mother left him, and I am sure he was glad to go... I still have the wonderful newspaper article about Dr. Ugo Fornari and what he did for the people of Ukerewe... May he now rest in eternal peace.

It was only fairly recently that I realised that Sister Pauline is not indestructible, when she sent me this message:

... I am still in Nyakato, and happy to be here. The pace of life suits me well. I did go away for 3 weeks to Sydney... After 3 weeks there I went to Kolkata, supposedly to 'see Loreto', but by the 3rd day there my lungs couldn't take the climate: humidity ... I ended up in the ICU for several days, then more days recuperating in Loreto. One of our Kenyan sisters who is a nurse, came to bring me back to Nairobi. Eventually I got back to Nyakato, where the climate is just right and I have fully recovered. What an experience.
    Love,
    (Sr) Pauline.

I checked up on her when Covid 19 struck.

How kind of you to write, dear Paola. I have thought of you often each time Brussels comes up in the news, and wonder where you

are taking your one-walk-a-day... Here in Mwanza, we have not felt the impact of the Lockdown which has so paralysed Kenya and Uganda, but schools have been closed for the past month...
   (Sr) Pauline

That's Sister Pauline. Strong, determined, committed, boundlessly energetic, and always looking outwards. My friend for ever. Will we meet again? And will I get to swim in her pool?

KILIMANJARO

1972-2001

Uhuru

December 1972
I was on a high. I'd just received my 'A' level results, and ahead of me lay what seemed like endless months of rest and fun before facing university. And I was setting off to climb Kilimanjaro with my father, my brother-in-law Gino, and four other Italian men. *This is the life*, I thought.

My father climbed Mount Kilimanjaro nine times over the course of twelve years, organising expeditions for Italian friends living in Dar. If you asked him why, he'd say, with his typical false modesty, 'It's my annual medical check-up.' But it was clear to us that he was compelled to prove himself, again and again. On three occasions, my mother joined the group.

He compared climbing Kilimanjaro with childbirth. '… a beautiful experience, but a gruelling one, at the end of which every climber without exception, with the little breath left in them, will say, "Never again". Just like almost every one of the mothers of the 5,000 babies I helped bring into the world.' Then he'd add, with a wry smile, 'Pain, exhaustion and anguish are soon forgotten.'

'Mountain of greatness'; 'mountain we failed to climb'; 'mountain of caravans': there are many theories as to what the name Kilimanjaro means. 'Mountain of whiteness' is the most common explanation, from the Swahili *'kilima'*, meaning 'hill', and the local tribal Chagga language *'njaro'*, which roughly translates as 'whiteness'. But the whiteness is nearly gone; about eighty per cent of the snow and ice has disappeared in the last hundred years, and scientists predict that there will be none left by 2040.

Kilimanjaro is more than a 'hill': situated just inside the Tanzania border with Kenya, it's the highest mountain in Africa, and the highest freestanding mountain in the world. Two of its three volcanic cones, Mawenzi and Shira, are extinct: they are linked by a long 'saddle' to the highest, dormant cone, Kibo, which soars above the surrounding savannah to an altitude of 5,895 metres.

The Marangu route, which is not technically difficult, starts at about 1,800 metres, and takes five days and four nights. Each climbing group is accompanied by a guide, an assistant guide, a cook, and porters who carry climbers' clothes and equipment, and the food that will be prepared along the way. Climbers carry a small backpack with a packed lunch and water.

This was the first of my father's climbs. Day One took us on gentle upward slopes through coffee and banana plantations and into the rainforest, where we spotted colobus monkeys, their long white feathery tails and capes sparkling in the dappled light as they swung from tree to tree. It was warm: we wore shorts, T-shirts, hats and simple sneakers, and carried a stick. Our first stop was Mandara Hut, 2,700 metres above sea level. This was a similar height to the summits of Mount Longonot in Kenya, and Monte Amaro in Abruzzo, both of which I had climbed.

The ever-cheerful porters, who had arrived long before us, welcomed us with a campfire and their Kilimanjaro song, which they sang in harmony, drumming on large saucepans:

Kilimanjaro, Kilimanjaro, Kilimanjaro,
Kilimanjaro mlima mrefu sana,

Na Mawenzi, na Mawenzi, na Mawenzi,
Na Mawenzi, mlima mrefu sana ...

(Kilimanjaro is a very high mountain; Mawenzi is a very high mountain.)

Glowing with sunburn and pride, I settled down to the first of many smoky, tough, delicious stews. This is doable, I thought after dinner, collapsing onto my hard bunk, tired from the seven-hour climb, adrenalin pounding through my veins.

Just as I was dropping off to sleep, my father walked into the hut and whispered, 'Have you washed your feet?' Feet? Clean feet were hardly my priority.

Ever since I can remember, my father regularly checked our feet once we were in bed, sending us off to the bathroom to scrub them if they didn't pass muster. I had thought I might be exempt up here.

Perhaps because he never raised it, my father's quiet voice always commanded respect. I struggled out of my damp sleeping bag, and wandered out into the cool air. I hardly needed my torch: above me, the magic carpet of the Milky Way swept through the sky, the Southern Cross clinging to it, lighting my way to the rudimentary washroom.

The next day, after a breakfast of strong tea and murky porridge, we climbed into alpine moorland, where the landscape was covered with giant lobelias and edelweiss. Seven hours and twelve kilometres later we reached Horombo hut, just below the saddle. We were now at 3,700 metres. The air was cool and crisp, but none of the group was suffering from altitude sickness... yet. Perhaps this was thanks to my father's mantra: 'If you feel you're going too slow, slow down.' This time I pre-empted my father and washed my feet in icy water before heading to my bunk.

It was on Day Three that fatigue and despondency set in. We hiked up a steep slope past the last few trees, and onto the barren, rocky moonscape of the relatively flat saddle. On our right loomed the craggy Mawenzi Peak. We turned left, facing the snowy Kibo Peak, which seemed to draw away further and further from us with every heavy step we took towards it. Just below the snowline, but far above the saddle, we could see Kibo Hut, our destination for today. We stopped at a sign that read 'Last Water' by a stream, drank, filled our bottles and plodded on, grateful in the knowledge that our porters had sufficient water supplies for the next day. The sketchy instructions we'd received at the mountain gate rang through my throbbing head: 'When you start vomiting blood, turn back.' I was pretty sure the park official had said 'when', not 'if'.

But somehow we made it up the slope at the end of the saddle to 4,500 metres and Kibo Hut. The fittest member of our group, an excellent tennis player in his thirties, was hit by severe mountain sickness and my father advised him not to continue. That evening we ate little. There was no singing and little chat. We took to our bunks early, dressed in our warmest climbing clothes. My father did not inspect my feet. The final ascent was to start at 1 a.m.; '... so you won't see the horror of what's facing you,' my father, who suffered from vertigo, joked. In fact, the reason for the early start is that the scree needs to be frozen so that you don't slide too much.

At midnight we were woken for a light breakfast. The temperature was below freezing. My head was hammering and I didn't want to eat. This was no longer the breeze I had anticipated. The six of us set off, with our guide and assistant guide. After two hours of taking three steps forwards and sliding two back, I realised I was alone with our assistant guide.

'Come,' he said, dragging me by the hand. 'They are waiting just above. Look.' In the beam of his torch I could see the zigzag path leading steeply upwards towards a cluster of lights.

At last I reached the others, who were sheltering at 5,150 metres in the Hans Meyer Cave, named after the first European to have reached the summit of Kilimanjaro, in 1889.

'I can't go on,' I croaked.

I wish my father had said, 'You can do this, just get on with it.' Instead he said, 'You've done well.' This was his first experience of high altitudes: he didn't want to take any risks.

*

December 1974
Willie and I rested in the Hans Meyer Cave with our guide. Almost a year after we had met at Edinburgh University, he had come home to Tanzania with me for the Christmas break.

'We can do this,' he whispered through his icy beard, and I believed him. Our objective was to reach Gilman's Point, on the crater's edge. In those days few people continued around the crater for three more hours, to the highest point, Uhuru Peak.

One tiny step at a time, often slipping backwards, we zigzagged up the mountain. As dawn broke to our right, bathing the surrounding glaciers in an incandescent gold, we stepped onto the rim of the crater. Leaning on our sticks, we gazed at the yellow lettering on the wooden sign which read 'You are now at Gilman's Point, 5,681 metres above sea level. Welcome and congratulations.' And in unison, we clutched our stomachs, leant over, and threw up in the pristine snow.

'Enough,' the guide said, smiling and puffing at a cigarette. 'You have made it.' And we have certificates to prove it.

*

January 1977
I lay in the snow at Gilman's Point.

'Just leave me here,' I mumbled to Christina. 'This is enough. You go on.' By this stage, my father, who by now had made it to Uhuru Peak several times, had discovered the altitude sickness medication, Diamox, and carefully dosed it out preventively. I wasn't suffering from nausea or headaches; I was simply exhausted.

Christina's family had a coffee farm on the lower slopes of the mountain, but she had never before attempted the climb. We were both in our final year at university. She had been my closest friend during my last years at boarding school. When we were teenagers, she often travelled the five hundred kilometres between her home and mine on the 'Luxury Bus' during the holidays, to enjoy the seaside and bright lights of Dar.

Christina looked down at me. 'No way. I'm not leaving you behind. I have spent three days getting this far, and this is it. Never again. You are getting up and you are coming with me to Uhuru Peak.'

Like my father, Christina spoke quietly, and her voice demanded attention. I struggled to my feet.

Three hours later, we hugged at Uhuru Peak, 5,895 metres above sea level. In a cairn there was a book for us to sign. At the front were written the words Julius Nyerere had spoken in 1959, when he was looking forward to the fulfilment of his dream of an independent Tanganyika: *'We, the people of Tanganyika, would like to light a candle and put it on the top of Mount Kilimanjaro. It will shine beyond our borders giving hope where there was despair, love where there was hate, and dignity where before there was only humiliation.'* Two Tanganyikan climbers had placed the book there on 9th December 1961, when the country had achieved independence. It was then that the peak was named Uhuru, which in Swahili means freedom.

Christina was the best climbing partner I could have hoped for: without her steady step ahead of me, I would never have continued. I will be eternally grateful to her, for showing me that the apparently impossible is achievable.

With tears flowing down my cheeks, I looked down over the plains glowing in the rosy dawn and wondered what the future could possibly hold for me, after this.

*

In 1981, when I was pregnant with our second child, Willie joined one of my father's climbs and reached Uhuru Peak.

In 2001, we waited together nervously at the mountain gate for our three children, aged sixteen, nineteen, and twenty-one, and cried tears of joy as we saw them emerge from the forest with triumphant smiles on their sunburnt faces: all of them had reached Uhuru Peak.

EDINBURGH

1973-1974

The Yellow Brick Road

It was miserable. Damp fog blanketed the black city, hugging to it the spicy, earthy smell of hops. The cold burrowed into my bones through necklines, cuff ends, and buttonholes. One evening I found myself getting into pyjamas at five o'clock: it had been dark for so long that I felt it must be bedtime.

Day after day I floated about, a rudderless boat trying to navigate from a lecture hall in one building to a tutorial in another, asking myself what someone as inadequate as I was doing attending one of the best universities in the world. I felt alone amongst thousands of students, all of whom looked confident and competent.

Why was I here in Edinburgh? I had sailed through 'A' levels by choosing subjects that came easily to me. Of the twenty-five girls in my year, about half got university entry grades. A university degree was the next logical step in our lives. We pored over prospectuses in the library, with little advice from our teachers.

My parents had no clear expectations of me, but were proud that I had done well. 'Try for Oxford or Cambridge,' they said. No, too much like hard work, too snobby, I told them. 'It has to be Edinburgh then,' they said. 'Papà loved studying there.' Okay, at least I knew where Edinburgh was. I had no ambition, no direction, and no drive. My mother went on about meeting the right man and getting a *lavoretto*.

By now I knew all about *lavoretti* and quite enjoyed them. School had ended in December 1972 and university was to start the following October: I spent the ten intervening months typing up translations on my mother's old Olivetti, and working as a guide for a tour company, driving Italian tourists to and from the airport in my father's Ford Cortina, accompanying them on trips out to islands, and ensuring they had a good time. The feeling of earning my own money was overwhelmingly satisfying, and I was brimming with self-assurance. But I knew these 'little jobs' did not constitute a viable future.

My application to do a Joint Honours Master's in Italian and French at Edinburgh University was successful, and I arrived in Scotland full of confidence. I chose English as a subsidiary subject. But after one tutorial during which a fellow student spouted intelligently about obscure metaphysical aspects of John Donne's poetry, I ditched it. We had barely touched poetry at school. Donne was a far cry from *Jane Eyre*, *Hamlet*, and *Sons and Lovers*. I realised this was not going to be as easy as I thought. I took up Linguistics instead: what a relief to find that no one seemed to know more than I did about the subject, and there was plenty of scope for creativity (or bluff?) with my knowledge of Swahili and a couple of Romance languages.

I was ignorant about politics, conscious of sounding English amongst my Scottish course mates, and I didn't fit in with any particular group. Soon my self-assurance started withering away, and I began to withdraw.

One evening I was caught up with a crowd who were smoking dope. A Portuguese student accosted me a little over-enthusiastically. I ran off, shaken and sobbing, and fortunately bumped into someone I vaguely knew. Seeing my state, he took me back to my hall of residence on the back of his motorbike.

My parents had booked me into the all-girl East Suffolk Road Halls, presided over by a tall and gangly woman called Miss Thin. You had to sign in and out, note all phone calls in a register, and dress up occasionally to sit at the High Table for dinner. It was a safe retreat, rather like boarding school.

The end of my first term couldn't come soon enough: sea, sand and regular sunrises and sunsets awaited me at home in Dar.

'I'm not going back,' I said to my parents. I felt justified in this decision: four years earlier Silvia had decided to quit Manchester University after one term. They listened to my woes, and cajoled me, telling me I should give it another chance. Silvia, after all, had had a good reason: her fiancé was in Dar and her future was lined up. I thought about it. Indeed, perhaps they were right: lolling about on the beach for the rest of my life was hardly an option.

'But I have to write an essay!' I complained, clutching at my last straw. 'In Italian. I can't do it. I can't go back if I haven't done my homework!'

'Of course you can write an essay,' my mother said. 'I'll help you. What's it about?'

'It's on the role of women in Italo Svevo's *La Coscienza di Zeno*.'

'I haven't read that,' my mother said. 'What's the plot?'

'Well, Zeno's a man who wants to give up smoking. He tries in various ways and eventually meets a doctor who tells him to write his thoughts in a diary. The book is the diary.'

'What women are in the book?'

I told my mother a bit about Zeno's wife, his sisters-in-law, and the relationships between them all. She asked me to fill in a few more details.

'Okay,' she said. 'Get a pen and paper. Start writing.' And without once going back on herself, only pausing when I interrupted with comments like 'Mamma, can you use a simpler word? One I would use? I would never write *atteggiamento materno*...' she dictated 'my' first ever essay written in Italian.

With no excuses left, sunburnt, rested, but unenthusiastic, I returned to Edinburgh, and was awarded an 'A' for my assignment.

The euphoria of the high grade soon wore off, and I retreated into my shell.

One evening – it was 19th January 1974 – a friend persuaded me to go to a party with her at one of the modern – and mixed – Pollock Halls of Residence, where she lodged, at the foot of Arthur's Seat. So, wearing a mauve long-sleeved T-shirt and beige brushed cotton jeans, I ditched my shoes in her room (it was cool not to wear shoes, I thought… I couldn't dance in shoes anyway and I'd lose them if I took them off), and she and I went off to Ewing Hall. I was grateful for the cover provided by the dark, jam-packed room and the smoky air.

*

In those days, young people danced in couples: usually a girl and a boy together, and occasionally, two girls, perhaps seeking to attract attention. People didn't dance alone, or in groups. There'd be a set of fast songs, followed by a set of slow ones. Between the fast and the slow, if either party said 'Thank you', that was it. If neither did, things turned promising.

Leaning against a wall, I looked around the musty room. In the penumbra, slouched in a chair in a corner, was a tall, strongly-built young man, smoking a pipe. He had shoulder-length, wavy hair. Why was someone so gorgeous alone? Why was he looking so miserable?

I took a deep breath and wound my way towards him. 'Will you dance?'

He turned his face towards me and smiled broadly. In the low light, above his green army jumper, I noticed slightly uneven teeth (rugby, I later learnt) and piercing blue eyes. And a few moments later we were on the dance floor. When the fast set ended, neither of us said 'Thank you'.

As we swayed to Elton John's 'Yellow Brick Road', a girl beside me called, 'My contact lens! It's fallen out!'

Without hesitating (I was a contact lens wearer and understood the gravity of the situation), I disengaged myself and hunted for the light switch. When I turned on the light, there was a collective groan from the heaving couples on the dance floor. I scrabbled on the floor and soon found the lens. The lights dimmed again.

After the party, the ground was cold and wet, and he carried all forty-five kilos of me to his hall across the road and up five flights of stairs to his room. I read the name on the door. William Hanna.

'I like your surname,' I said.

We talked. His voice was soft, his accent musical. He told me he was from Belfast. I knew a little about Northern Ireland: at school we had prayed for the people caught up in The Troubles, which, according to my nuns, were all about Catholics being oppressed by Protestants. His father was a minister, he said, and I understood that was like a pastor, which made him a Protestant. He explained the Northern Irish situation to me, and told me he had come to Edinburgh to escape it, and because his father had studied there. He was studying French with European Law: he believed in the European dream. We realised we were already attending lectures together.

He read a passage from Robert Louis Stevenson's *Edinburgh*.

I told him about my family and my home, and was surprised that not only did he know where Dar was; he was interested in my life there. He says I had an 'outrageously mahogany tan' and blonde streaks in my hair. Exotic. He liked my 'spontaneity' over the contact lens. (I thought it was common sense.)

His girlfriend had ditched him the previous evening, and he'd lost his rugby match that afternoon. I'm not sure which event had upset him more, but he now seemed to be recovering.

'See you at the lecture on Monday,' he said at the end of the evening.

I spent Sunday thinking about him. I realised he was many things I wasn't. Focussed and grounded, he had an idea of where he was going. And it didn't take me long to realise that wherever that may be, I wanted to go with him...

On Monday, outside the lecture theatre, I scoured the three hundred girls and thirty boys gathered at the door. I later learnt that he had just been to the cafeteria with his ex-girlfriend, who had wanted to finalise things on a friendly note. She was still hanging about nearby, and must have witnessed me as I spotted him, called out 'Hey, Willie!' rushed through the crowd, and leapt off my feet into his arms, straddling my legs around his waist.

'Spontaneous,' he says, forty-eight years later.

'Common sense,' I reply.

ROME

November 2021

Closure

When I was thirty, I had a dream, which is as clear in my mind now as it was then. My father was sixty at the time, but in my dream, he was stooped, wrinkled, and old. He sat on a wooden chair, leaning forwards onto a walking stick. He called together Enrico, Silvia and me.

'You know that I don't believe in God,' he said. 'But when I am gone, I will live on, in you three.'

*

November 2021
Arm in arm, Enrico in the middle, we walk down the road from my parents' apartment, passing familiar shops, Bangladeshi clothes stalls, overflowing rubbish containers, the post office and the metro station. The day is grey, wet, and windy. How many times have we covered these few hundred metres in the thirty-six years since my parents returned from Africa? Hundreds, but rarely together.

Round the corner, opposite the pharmacy and beside the newspaper kiosk, we reach the taxi stand and approach a cab.

'No,' the driver snaps. 'Can't take three of you. Covid measures.'

'But we're one family!' Silvia says.

'No: rules are rules,' a second driver replies. 'You must take two cabs.'

We look at each other in despair. I feel my eyes moistening.

Our father died in February, two and a half years after our mother. At last, after nine months of typical Italian red tape and confusion, today is the day we have been summoned to scatter his ashes at the Garden of Remembrance in Rome's largest crematorium, where my mother's ashes lie.

'I'll take you all,' a third taxi driver says. 'They're talking nonsense. Jump in.'

'Titch in the middle,' Enrico says. Obviously. I know my place. And take it. Silvia and Enrico ooze confidence; I am convinced something will go wrong, and sob all the way to the crematorium. Rain spatters the windscreen. 'They're with us,' Silvia whispers, looking out of her window up into the clouds.

An hour later, we are at the crematorium, walking through the garden. The rain has stopped, the sky is clear. Silvia cradles the urn. We reach a fountain. The ashes are poured into the water and disappear through a funnel into the earth below. Feeling a weight lifted off my shoulders, I remember the prayer we used to say at school: *Remember, man, that thou art dust, and into dust thou shalt return.*

*

It seemed a miracle that in the midst of the Covid pandemic Enrico was able to travel from Pietra Ligure in Liguria, Silvia from Houston, and I from Brussels. Both Enrico and Silvia were recovering from serious illnesses. Particularly for Silvia, who had recently undergone a major operation, this was a feat. We had no particular plan of action, but we had an objective: to spend twelve days clearing my parents' apartment so as to put it up for sale. We hadn't spent so much time together in the last fifty years since boarding school holidays.

Though fate had scattered us around the world, all of us had travelled to Rome as often as we could, especially in recent years. For years my father – and, until she died, my mother – had been supported by their devoted Filipino carers, Benny and Lori. From the start of the pandemic, we had videocalls with my father every Sunday evening. Enrico and his son Luca were with him when he died, and after that, we continued our Sunday sibling calls.

My parents were of the generation that never threw anything away: every shelf and cupboard was stacked with trinkets, neatly labelled letters, negatives, school reports, newspaper cuttings, and albums filled with black and white photos. Pictures and portraits adorned every wall. As we studied each item, we experienced a condensed fast replay of our family's life, from before we were born, through our childhood years and into our adulthood. We felt our father's struggles as he forged his career in rural Abruzzo, and followed his 'leap into the light' as he took his young family to Tanganyika. We relived all our moves from one village to the next, and our boarding school days, through the colonial period and on to independence. I cringed every time I caught sight of the shell collection, a set of ivory tusks, and two turtle shells. Photos took us back to our parents' move back to Rome when they retired after over three decades in Africa. How must that have been for them? They did what they could to continue their lives dedicated to others. For as long as was possible, my father continued practising as a doctor at the San Gallicano hospital, seeing immigrant patients who had no right to medical care, and my mother worked at the Caritas soup kitchen.

Examining each item was sometimes joyful, sometimes painful. Tears flowed as we watched our parents' two armchairs being taken away: they had sat there side by side for over a decade, as my mother slowly withdrew into the mysterious world inside her head. 'It's a privilege to be able to rest beside her,' my father wrote to us two years before she died, 'listening to her breath, feeling her pulse beating in unison with mine, and returning the squeeze of her hand.' And when she'd gone, he continued sitting in his armchair, reading aloud from his favourite book, Cesare Pascarella's *La Scoperta dell'America*, a spoof on Columbus' voyage to the New World, which perhaps took him back to the adventures of his youth. His carers regularly sent us videos of him reading.

We soon got used to each other's styles. Enrico took quick decisions, and knew what he wanted. Silvia was selective. She needed time. She needed space. She needed to be left alone. But she was systematic and got results. I was somewhere in the middle... inconsistent but enthusiastic.

Throughout those intense twelve days, we had the constant quiet support of our families. When the time came for us to take our three separate ways, our mission had been accomplished. Furniture, kitchenware, trinkets, books and all the shells had been distributed to cousins, friends, and strangers, and the flat was empty and on the market. Three shipments were on the way to our homes.

The ivory tusks are now with Enrico in Liguria. The fossilised trunk from our Garden Avenue house in Dar is with Silvia in Houston. The family table, pieced together from the Kinondoni Road house, is in my Edinburgh kitchen.

*

As we sit in the taxi on the way home from the crematorium, I feel an emptiness: it's too quiet. 'But where's the thunder?' I ask. 'We need thunder!' And just as I finish speaking, dark clouds gather above us, a distant rumble gradually rolls towards us, and the heavens open.

'They're there,' I say. 'They're with us.' And clutching hands, we look up into the anthracite sky.

Glossary

(Swahili words, except where otherwise specified)

Askari:	soldier, guard
Banda:	thatched hut
Banghi:	marijuana
Bilauri:	glass
Bravi ragazzi (*Italian*):	good kids
Bwana Mganga:	traditional doctor, medicine man
Dagaa:	type of small fish
Daktari:	doctor
Dawa:	medicine
Dhobi:	laundryman
Duka:	shop
Dudu:	insect
Embe:	mango
Fupi:	short
Hodi/Karibu:	May I come in?/Welcome
Kanga:	brightly-coloured cloth wrapper
Kikapu:	basket
Kopje (*Afrikaans*):	hillock

Magaro (*Italian*):	local witchdoctor
Mzungu (*pl. wazungu*):	white person
Ngalawa:	traditional double outrigger canoe
Panga:	machete
Papai:	pawpaw
Pole:	I empathise with your suffering
Rafiki:	friend
Safi (*kisafi*):	clean
Salaam Alaikum:	Peace to you (Moslem greeting)
Shamba:	cultivated plot of ground
Shikamoo/Marahaba:	respectful greeting and response (lit. Touching your leg/Accepting your respect)
Sice:	groom (for horses)
Ten centi:	cheap cigarette (literally ten cents)
Treccine d'oro (*Italian*):	golden plaits
Tutaonana:	See you later

Acknowledgements

Many people helped me during the writing of this book, by commenting on the original blog version, reading extracts, giving tips, and jogging my memory. I would like to thank Alyson Hilbourne, Anna Gadola, Bess Stonehouse; my fellow-members of the Itinerant Writers' Club, particularly Helen Moat and Moira Ashley; and alumni of Loreto Msongari and St. Mary's, especially Alison Holmes, Anna Capitani, Christina Willink, Marta Fiorotto, Val Hookings, Jerry Bary, and all those who sent me their testimonies of the Congo refugee crisis.

Through the blog, I came into contact with many people from my family's early days in Abruzzo and Tanganyika: my thanks go out to Anna Stack, Cristina DeThomasis, David Plater, Geraldine Hayes-Jones, John Goodman, José Lamb, Jenny Mattingly, Linda Scipione, Roger Wooller, Steve Deane, and Tom Syratt, for sharing their stories. Many relatives got in touch when they heard about the project: thank you, Anna Dolci, Marco Elli, Rita Cossa, and Rosaria de Peniche.

I am grateful to Jonathan Lamb for allowing me to use a verse from his poem 'The Ugly Baby'; and to dear Sisters Caitriona, Germaine and Pauline for approving what I have written about them. Bill Osborne enhanced every photo in the book: thanks, Bill. Thanks to my husband Willie for encouraging me to take on this project, helping me over the hurdles, and giving me confidence; to my children for their support; and to my brother Enrico and sister Silvia who held me by the hand all the way.

And thanks to my friend and editor Nicola Wood, who meticulously went through the manuscript, made pertinent suggestions and offered valuable advice.

References

Carlo Levi, *Christ Stopped at Eboli*, Penguin Modern Classics, 2020 (original Italian version, *Cristo si è fermato a Eboli*, published in 1945 by Grassano)

Henry Morton Stanley, *How I Found Livingstone in Central Africa*, Dover Publications, 2002 (originally published in 1871 by Scribner, Armstrong & Co)

Jonathan Lamb, *The Ugly Baby*, Poor Tree Press, 2007

This book is printed on paper from sustainable sources managed under the Forest Stewardship Council (FSC) scheme.

It has been printed in the UK to reduce transportation miles and their impact upon the environment.

For every new title that Matador publishes, we plant a tree to offset CO_2, partnering with the More Trees scheme.

MORE TREES
LET'S PLANT A BILLION TREES

For more about how Matador offsets its environmental impact, see www.troubador.co.uk/about/